THE COMPLETE HEALTHY EATING COOKBOOK

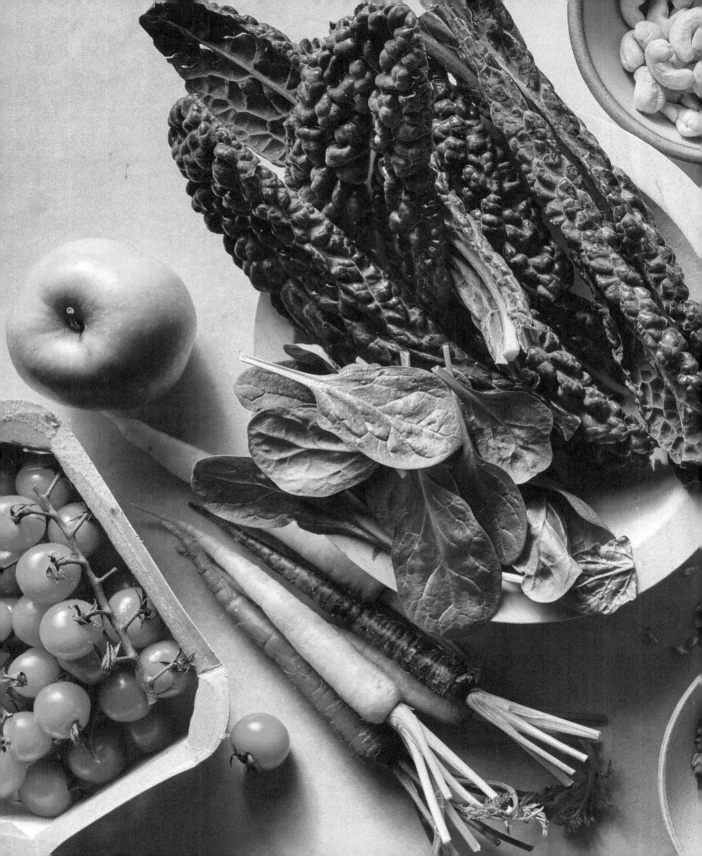

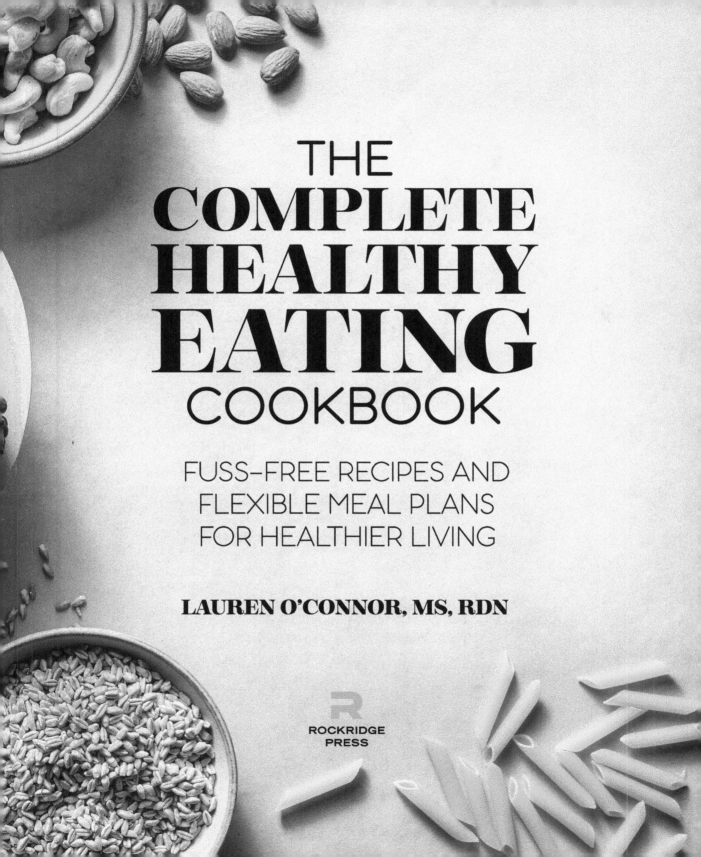

THE
COMPLETE
HEALTHY
EATING
COOKBOOK

FUSS-FREE RECIPES AND FLEXIBLE MEAL PLANS FOR HEALTHIER LIVING

LAUREN O'CONNOR, MS, RDN

ROCKRIDGE
PRESS

For general information on our other products and services or to obtain technical support, please contact our Customer Care Department within the United States at (866) 744-2665, or outside the United States at (510) 253-0500.

Rockridge Press publishes its books in a variety of electronic and print formats. Some content that appears in print may not be available in electronic books, and vice versa.

TRADEMARKS: Rockridge Press and the Rockridge Press logo are trademarks or registered trademarks of Callisto Media Inc. and/or its affiliates, in the United States and other countries, and may not be used without written permission. All other trademarks are the property of their respective owners. Rockridge Press is not associated with any product or vendor mentioned in this book.

Interior and Cover Designer: Angela Navarra
Art Producer: Sue Bischofberger
Editor: Reina Glenn

Photography © 2021 Antonis Achilleos; food styling by Rishon Hanners.

ISBN: Print 978-1-64876-624-4
eBook 978-1-64876-123-2
R0

I'D LIKE TO DEDICATE THIS BOOK TO MY HUSBAND, JP, FOR
BEING MY PARTNER IN HEALTH AND HAPPINESS.

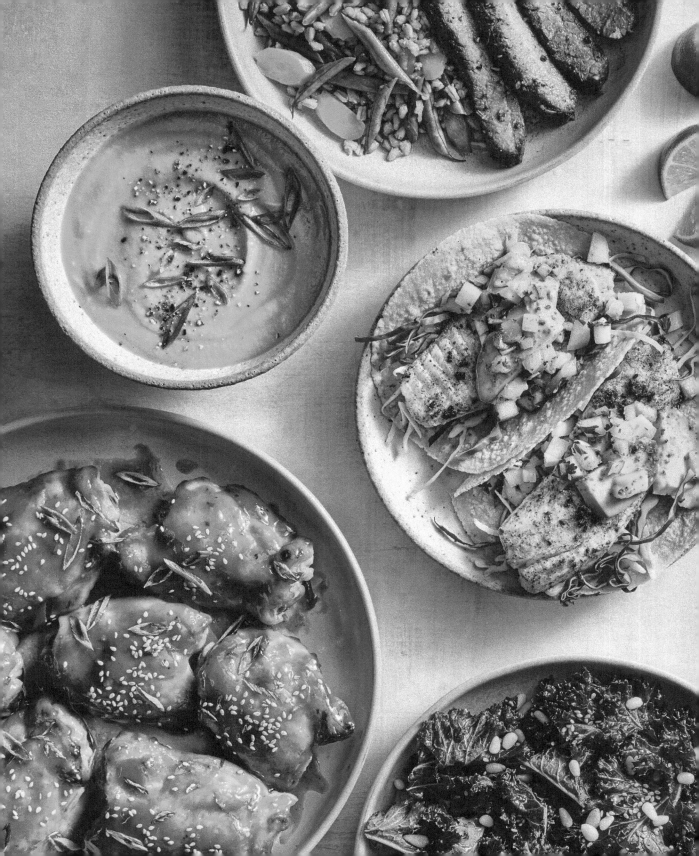

CONTENTS

INTRODUCTION   viii

CHAPTER 1: HEALTHY EATING FROM START TO FINISH   1

CHAPTER 2: HEALTHY MEAL PLANS   19

CHAPTER 3: BREAKFASTS AND SMOOTHIES   33

CHAPTER 4: SOUPS, SALADS, AND SANDWICHES   51

CHAPTER 5: VEGAN/VEGETARIAN   69

CHAPTER 6: FISH AND SEAFOOD   95

CHAPTER 7: POULTRY   119

CHAPTER 8: PORK AND BEEF   149

CHAPTER 9: DESSERTS   175

CHAPTER 10: SNACKS, SIDES, AND STAPLES   189

MEASUREMENT CONVERSIONS   206

RESOURCES   207

REFERENCES   208

INDEX   210

INTRODUCTION

My health journey began years ago. I was young and college bound and had my whole life ahead of me. But I was also obsessed with being thin. Those last months in high school had me on edge; I wanted to be perfect, and part of that included my outer appearance. Years later, I discovered my anorexic tendencies were tied to control. I had mastered food restriction, but I was still low on confidence.

At my lowest point, I was 88 pounds and miserable, despite being lean. And although I successfully recovered, I still fought those demons surrounding food. I suffered bouts of self-restriction during the years that followed. It was a spiral that kept me from truly enjoying life, especially during major festivities.

Eventually, I learned I could enjoy tasty foods without fearing weight gain. I discovered that balance, variety, and "listening to my body" played important roles in healthy eating and overall happiness. I grew confident that I could help others who had suffered just like me. I went on to get my master's degree in nutritional science. My career path was born.

As a registered dietitian, I have helped hundreds of people build a positive relationship with food while supporting their health needs. My focus is now on digestive disorders, including acid reflux/GERD, but my philosophy remains the same. Food is meant to be enjoyed, not restricted, and although healthy eating is important, it has to be delicious, too.

You may have heard this before, but it's absolutely worth mentioning again: healthy eating is about changing your habits for the long term. You can't rely on a quick fix—it simply isn't sustainable!

Crash dieting, restriction, and "detoxing" affect your energy and mood and can even lead to nutrient deficiencies. While some people must avoid certain foods for medical reasons, it is my goal to loosen restrictions where I can and open the door for a delicious variety of foods to suit those individual needs.

The goal of this book is to make healthy eating realistic, accessible, and absolutely delicious. You won't be spending excess time or effort in the kitchen, nor will eating this way require a lot of money. You can count on the recipes to keep you satisfied. But most importantly, they will help you build a healthy lifestyle that you can enjoy.

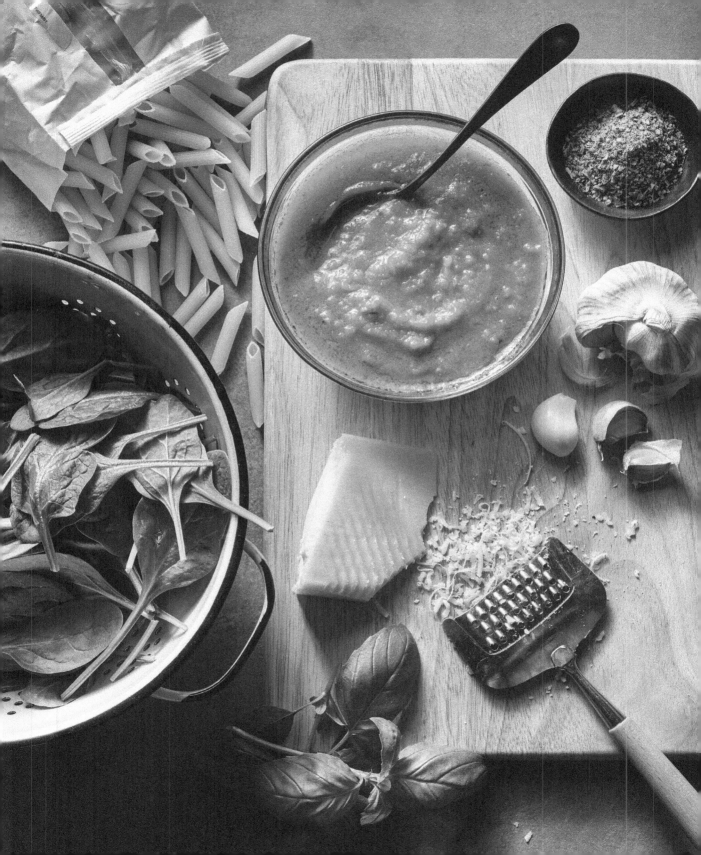

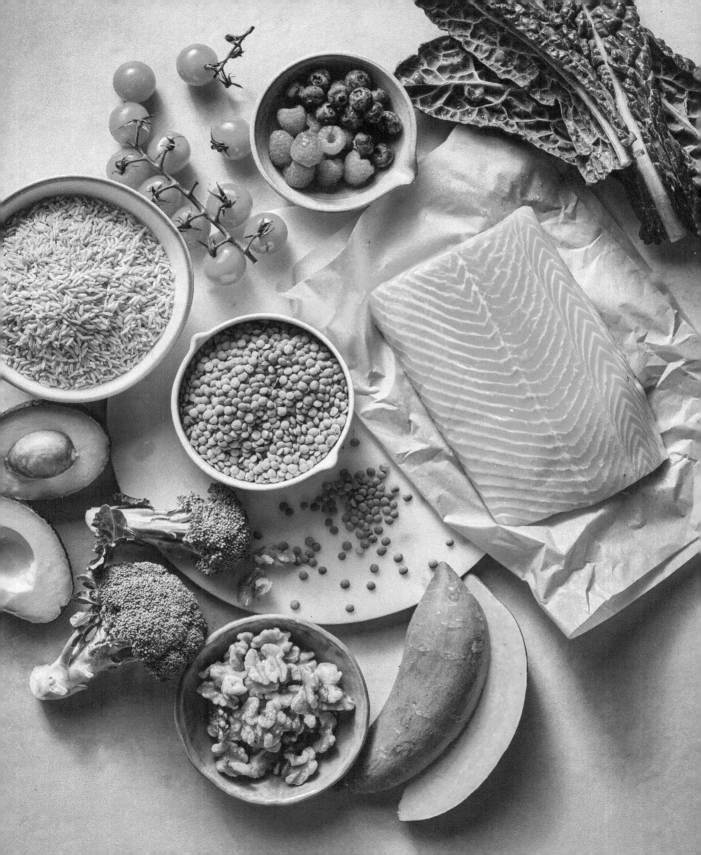

CHAPTER 1

HEALTHY EATING FROM START TO FINISH

Healthy eating can be colorful, enticing, and absolutely divine. Building your plate with fruits and vegetables creates a rainbow of possibilities. This book has a variety of ways to feature fruits and veggies in your meals, from smoothies, soups, and stir-fries to colorful sides. You'll also find juicy chicken, glazed pork, seared fish, and plenty of tasty vegetarian alternatives.

This book provides simple, effective methods of cooking to enhance the flavors of naturally healthy foods using homemade sauces, dressings, and carefully selected herbs for a mouthwatering finish and presentation.

With 30-minute meals to accommodate your busy schedule, family-friendly options, and a variety of dishes to suit vegan, vegetarian, or gluten-free needs, this book is your all-in-one guide to healthy eating.

DEFINING HEALTHY IN 1, 2, 3

Healthy eating can be defined in a variety of ways. From the Mediterranean diet and DASH protocol to the USDA's MyPlate, you'll find that the common theme is a focus on mostly plant-based whole foods. Not just fruits and veggies but also whole grains, legumes, herbs and spices, and healthy fats from nuts and seeds. There's even some wiggle room for added sugars, albeit in limited amounts. Consider the following your basic rules for eating healthy.

EAT WHOLE (UNPROCESSED) FOODS

Whole foods are those foods you consume that appear closest to their origins—think brown rice, oats, almonds, canned beans, kale, apples, chicken, fish, beef, milk, and eggs. Although some whole foods are milled, canned, ground, or minimally preserved for safety and freshness, the processing is minor.

Highly processed foods are the foods you should limit. If you aren't sure whether a food is processed, just look at the label. There will likely be some ingredients you don't recognize. Look out for and avoid partially hydrogenated oils (trans fats), added sugars or alternative sweeteners, artificial flavorings, and dyes. These additives often counteract the nutritional value of these foods. Yes, bologna offers protein, but whole-food protein, such as lean pork, is a better option. We'll get more into the specifics later in this chapter.

BALANCE YOUR PLATE

Your ideal plate consists mainly of plant-based foods. The USDA's Dietary Guidelines for Americans suggest a plant-forward approach because research suggests that your best health is associated with higher consumption of plant foods and fewer animal proteins, though beef, pork, and poultry can certainly fit within a healthy diet.

Whether you choose an animal or a plant source for your protein, you'll be portioning your meal so that one-quarter of your plate is filled with lean protein, another quarter of your plate is filled with complex (fiber-rich) carbs, and the remaining half of your plate is filled with non-starchy vegetables—including some healthy fats such as nuts, seeds, avocado, and olive oil.

To give you an idea of how this might look, here's an example of a heart-healthy plate:

CHICKEN QUINOA SALAD

→ Non-starchy vegetable (half of the plate): spinach or other dark leafy green
→ Lean protein (one-quarter of the plate): 3 to 4 ounces chopped boneless, skinless chicken breast
→ Complex carb (one-quarter of the plate): ⅓ to ½ cup quinoa
→ Additions: 2 tablespoons crumbled low-fat feta or nuts and/or seeds (or a combo of both), 1 to 2 teaspoons olive oil, squeeze of lemon juice

MIND YOUR PORTIONS

There are countless negative consequences to habitual overeating, including sluggishness, slowed metabolism, and increased risk for heart disease. Portioning your meals and snacks is a good first step toward a healthier you.

The beauty of portion sizing is that it fits so well within the guidelines for a balanced plate. Sticking to ½ cup of brown rice and 3 to 4 ounces of fish leaves plenty of room to fill the remaining half of your plate with vegetables (aim for at least 1 cup). Individual needs may vary when it comes to overall intake, but this is a good rule of thumb for balancing your plate.

This book focuses on building a balanced plate by choosing high-quality foods, including a wide variety of fruits and vegetables, lean proteins, whole grains, and healthy fats while limiting dairy and added sugars. But just as importantly, it focuses on portion control.

Always listen to your body and check in with your healthcare provider, especially if you have a medical condition. Consult with a dietitian to help you tailor these guidelines to fit your specific needs.

LIFESTYLE CHANGES

Establishing a healthy eating pattern is a huge part of improving your health, but it's not the only thing you should master. How you function and feel also depends on your hydration, exercise, sleep, and stress management. Along with a healthy diet, these factors play a synergistic role in your overall health.

Hydration

Our bodies are close to 60 percent water. Our skin, brain, heart, and digestive organs depend on it. How well we hydrate has an effect on how we perform physically and mentally, too. Although individual needs may vary, eight (8-ounce) glasses of water per day is a reasonable goal, according to the Mayo Clinic. If you drink 1 to 2 glasses of water first thing in the morning, you'll be off to a good start.

Exercise

Get out of that chair and stretch those legs! It may help you refocus or reset when you've spent quite some time online. According to a 2018 study in *Frontiers in Public Health*, just 10 minutes of walking can have a positive effect on your mental acuity, so aim to take frequent computer breaks. Current World Health Organization guidelines recommend 150 to 300 minutes of moderate to intense aerobic activity per week. Breaking it down to 20- or 30-minute sessions can help keep your weekly exercise goal attainable.

Sleep

Sleep is your body's means of recharging, and it also plays a role in appetite control. A 2017 study from *Scientific Reports* found that lack of sleep throws your hormones out of whack, decreasing leptin (the hormone that keeps you satisfied) while increasing ghrelin (the hormone that signals hunger). Insufficient sleep may also raise your cortisol levels, increasing both your stress and appetite. This means you're more likely to overconsume when you've been sleep deprived. Tip: Plan quieter activities closer to bedtime and aim for eight hours of quality sleep by setting a reasonable lights-out time.

Stress Management

You may be doing everything else right, but if you aren't managing your stress, it can wreak havoc on your health. Stress has been linked to excess stomach acid and inflammation in the gut, according to a 2017 article in *EXCLI Journal*. Because extreme stress affects your digestion, it also affects your mood and how you function. Research has indicated that there is a connection between the brain and the gut. Learning to manage your stress through quieting activities such as reading, yoga, or even talking to a friend can help you manage those sparks before they go ablaze.

EAT BETTER, FEEL BETTER

Science links healthy eating habits to a reduced risk of chronic disease, but for those with existing health issues, healthy eating is even more imperative. Healing your gut, reducing inflammation, and increasing your energy are just a few reasons to stay on board.

GUT HEALTH

Consuming adequate amounts of fiber and probiotics supports gut health. Fiber keeps the digestive system running smoothly, and probiotics support a healthy gut environment. This book ensures that you meet your daily fiber needs by providing plenty of meals, snacks, sides, and even desserts that contain at least 3 grams of fiber (with many entrées providing 7 grams or more). Plus, many of the recipes also call for probiotic-rich ingredients, such as Greek yogurt.

AUTOIMMUNE/INFLAMMATION

Sugars and saturated fats can lead to inflammatory responses in the body. Saturated fats can raise cholesterol levels, particularly those types of lipoproteins (e.g., LDL cholesterol) that are considered harmful, according to a 2016 study from *Progress in Cardiovascular Diseases*. The researchers found that diets high in sugars raise blood sugar, impair insulin response, and significantly elevate the risk for heart disease. Consuming trans fats may increase the overall risk of premature death.

Inflammation in the body can manifest in pain, tightness, and digestive issues (bloating, nausea, cramps, etc.). A 2017 study showed that chronic inflammation increases the risk of heart disease and cancer, and it has also been linked to autoimmune disorders. By reducing excess sugars, trans fats, and saturated fats and eating nutrient-dense foods instead, you can lower your likelihood of developing such negative health issues.

This book provides a good variety of recipes that limit highly processed foods and focus on quality proteins, fiber-rich carbohydrates, and healthy fats that will help keep your body in check.

INCREASED ENERGY

Do you recall that weighed-down feeling from eating too much in one sitting? Overeating can zap your energy and make you feel fatigued for hours on end. By eating the right amount of the foods that support good health, you'll have the energy you need to function and feel good.

We get energy from food and also from movement. Exercise elicits those good-feeling endorphins and elevates your physical energy. So, when you include healthy eating and exercise, you get more bang for your buck!

WEIGHT LOSS

You can reduce your caloric intake without sacrificing taste or flavor, but minding your portions is key. Remember that a serving of protein is 3 to 4 ounces and a serving of carbs (choose high-fiber, a.k.a. complex, carbs) is just ½ cup and leave the remainder of your plate for non-starchy vegetables and a sprinkling of healthy fats.

This book's recipes are all designed to help you get the quality and balance of nutrients you need to stay healthy and satisfied.

YOUR NEW GO-TO INGREDIENTS

To keep things simple, you can divide healthy foods into three main categories: healthy fats, lean protein, and high-fiber carbs (which include starchy vegetables and fruits). As previously mentioned, these foods need to fit into a balanced plate so you can get all your essential nutrients. Healthy fats help with the metabolism and absorption of certain nutrients. Lean proteins support your muscles and bones, and those high-fiber carbs support your digestive needs. Together, the three main types of healthy foods keep your organs and systems running smoothly.

HEALTHY FATS

Healthy fats are composed mainly of unsaturated fats. They support your hair, skin, and nails, improving texture, strength, and elasticity. They also support your brain, which is made up of 60 percent fat, including EPA and DHA omega-3 fatty acids.

Research recognizes the importance of EPA (eicosapentaenoic acid) and DHA (docosahexaenoic acid) in supporting brain integrity and function, according to a 2018 review in *Nutrients*. These essential fatty acids also support the immune system. And as previously mentioned, all healthy fats help the body absorb fat-soluble nutrients, including vitamin D, which is necessary for strong bones and muscle health.

Healthy fat sources include walnuts, peanuts, cashews, almonds, nut butters, avocado, olive oil, and olives. Choose raw or roasted nuts (salted or unsalted)—skip the sweetened or seasoned varieties. Just be mindful that salt can add up, so when preparing your dishes, you may want to opt for unsalted varieties. Choose all-natural nut butters that contain only nuts and salt. You will often find oil separation in these types of butters, but you can easily stir them before use. If the nut butter becomes dried over time, adding a little oil won't hurt. When choosing olive oils, look for cold-pressed, canned, or jarred options.

Note: Dairy products do contain some healthy (unsaturated) fats, but much more of their fat content is saturated. Because of this, you will want to limit them in a healthy diet.

LEAN PROTEIN

Proteins are what we refer to as "the building blocks of life." Your cells, tissues, and organs are made up of proteins, which give them their structure and shape.

Lean protein comes from both plants and animals. You don't have to rely on just chicken, fish, pork, and eggs to serve your needs. Quinoa, tofu, lentils, and canned beans are excellent sources of plant-based protein; canned beans contain as much as 20 grams of protein per ½ cup serving. This book provides a variety of vegetarian options, from Veggie Meatloaf (page 86) to Sautéed Eggplant with Peppers and Onions (page 75). The latter recipe gets its protein from the combination of spinach, eggplant, sweet potato, bell peppers, and onions. But you don't have to pack tons of protein in all at once—a little here and there adds up, so you'll get plenty to meet your needs.

Lean animal proteins are much easier to quantify than plant-based proteins. For example, you can get about 20 grams of protein from 3 ounces of chicken. Good options include boneless, skinless chicken breasts and thighs. Look for cuts of beef or pork (or ground options) that are 80 to 85 percent lean (or 93 percent extra lean). Flank steak is an example of a lean cut of beef.

Organic, pasture-raised, non-GMO, and grass-fed animal proteins are quality choices. But if your budget is tight, these labels are not mandatory for ensuring health and safety. The government already has stringent guidelines for the use of antibiotics and the ways that poultry and cattle must be raised.

HIGH-FIBER CARBOHYDRATES

Carbohydrates are the natural sugars, starches, and fiber found in plant-based foods. They are an excellent source of energy—your brain's preferred source, in fact. High-fiber options are recommended because their fiber content helps you feel full and promotes healthy blood sugar levels.

A variety of plant foods contain soluble and insoluble fiber; soluble is great for cholesterol control, and insoluble is great for regular digestion. You won't need to worry about the specific amounts of each type of fiber if you consume plenty of different types of plant-based foods. Soluble sources of fiber include oats, beans, apples, and pears. Insoluble fiber, also found in beans, is found in wheat (pasta and whole-grain bread) and starchy vegetables, such as green beans and potatoes.

High-fiber carbohydrates contain 5 grams or more per serving. Because beans and legumes are already a rich source of fiber, you'll simply need to look for low-sodium canned varieties and be sure to rinse and drain them before using. However, when it comes to multigrain breads or crackers, you may find few options that contain 5 grams of fiber. So, choosing options with at least 3 grams of fiber per serving is just fine.

Fruits and starchy vegetables are also great ways to get in ample fiber. A medium pear contains 5 grams of fiber and a medium roasted sweet potato contains nearly 4 grams. When choosing your produce, organic is a great option. But if buying organic doesn't fit within your budget, washing your produce before cooking can help remove pesticides.

EAT	LIMIT	AVOID
FRUITS AND VEGETABLES	**DAIRY**	**PROCESSED SUGARS**
Apples, arugula, berries, broccoli, corn, green beans, kale, oranges, pears, russet potatoes, spinach, sweet potatoes, tomato*	Cow's milk, all varieties of cheese, flavored yogurts (choose low-fat options when consuming) Choosing low-fat cheese** instead of full-fat cheese means that you'll consume less saturated fat. Yogurt can be beneficial because of its probiotic content. Low-fat plain Greek yogurt is a healthy option in moderation.	It's easy to recognize cane sugar, but processed (or added) sugars come under many names, including: • caramel • dextrose • high-fructose corn syrup • invert sugar • maltose • molasses • rice syrup
WHOLE GRAINS AND LEGUMES	**ERYTHRITOL, MONK FRUIT, AND STEVIA**	**PROCESSED AND CURED MEATS**
Brown rice, buckwheat, chickpeas, farro, lentils, oats, peas, quinoa, soybeans, wild rice	These no-calorie sweeteners can help those with a sweet tooth prevent high blood sugars, but limiting is important. Excess consumption has been shown to cause bloating and gas.	Cured bacon, bologna, hot dogs, salami

*This is just a short list to get you started. All fruits and vegetables are recommended as long as you don't have an allergy or sensitivity.

**You can find low-fat versions of feta, cheddar, and Jack cheeses, and part-skim ricotta is also stocked in most grocery stores. Fresh mozzarella is lower in fat than most cheeses. If you choose a low-moisture mozzarella (e.g., packaged sandwich slices or shredded), you can find low-fat options. Thinly sliced deli cheese is a great option, because you'll still get the distribution of flavor but with fewer calories and less fat.

EAT	LIMIT	AVOID
LEAN POULTRY AND FISH	**RED MEATS**	**HIGH-SODIUM SAUCES AND CONDIMENTS**
Boneless, skinless chicken breasts or thighs; haddock; halibut; salmon***; tilapia; lean ground turkey; turkey breasts	Beef, lamb, pork, veal	Look for low-sodium sauces and condiments and be mindful of how much you use.
HEALTHY FATS	**HONEY AND MAPLE SYRUP**	**HIGHLY PROCESSED PACKAGED SNACKS AND SOFT DRINKS**
Almonds, avocado, cashews, olive oil, olives, peanuts, pistachios, pumpkin seeds, sunflower seeds, walnuts	Although these contain some trace nutrients, your body recognizes all forms of sugar in the same way.**** The intense sweetness of honey and maple syrup simply makes it easier to use less of these sweeteners.	Bars, chips, cookies, crackers, pretzels, soda of any kind (diet or regular)

***Though wild-caught salmon tends to be leaner, it can easily dry out if overcooked (even slightly). Farm-raised is still a healthy choice. Coho and Chum salmon are two of the leanest types of salmon you can find. Atlantic salmon and King salmon are fattier, but they also contain a greater amount of omega-3s.

****Whether you opt for table sugar or that which is derived from bees or trees (e.g., honey or maple syrup), limit your consumption. Excess sugar consumption can manifest in diabetic conditions and heart disease, according to a *JAMA Internal Medicine* study.

"HEALTHY" FOODS THAT ARE
ACTUALLY BAD FOR YOU

Can "healthy" foods be bad for you? Absolutely. Be wary of those product claims. In fact, most "diet" foods do not support your health because they are highly processed. This includes artificial sweeteners and "low-fat" products.

The 1980s were an era when "diet" foods reigned, replacing fat with refined carbs. But instead of whittling waistlines, it did the opposite. A 2018 study in *Clinical Chemistry* linked heightened consumption of refined carbs not only to weight gain but also to increased cholesterol and insulin resistance.

Removing such deceptively "healthy" foods is an easy way to start your health journey. In many cases, there's a healthier alternative to those processed foods you have grown to love. The following list provides healthy substitutions for common "diet" foods you are better off avoiding.

1. **Choose flavored seltzer or sparkling water, not diet soda.** Diet sodas are chock full of artificial sweeteners like aspartame, which are intensely sweet. Consuming too many artificially sweetened products may actually enhance the desire for sweetness (without regard to calories), ultimately resulting in increased appetite and weight gain. Some recent studies suggest that artificial sweeteners may also affect insulin sensitivity and contribute to diabetes, particularly in obese individuals. Flavored seltzer has no added sugar and still gives you that bubbly taste. Or you can simply add lemon or fresh mint to plain sparkling water.

2. **Choose plain yogurt, not a flavored variety.** Flavored yogurts contain added sugars, dyes, and artificial flavorings. Instead, flavor your yogurt with natural whole foods such as wild blueberries, raspberries, or a combo of mixed berries—you'll get the benefits of fiber and antioxidants, too.

3. **Choose homemade smoothies over "diet" shakes.** Sure, "diet" shakes are convenient and promise appetite control, but they often include chemicals, added sugars, artificial sweeteners, and other highly processed ingredients that don't serve you nutritionally. To get you started, this book provides tasty, simple smoothie recipes including Strawberry-Basil Smoothie (page 41) and Mango Cream Smoothie (page 43).

4. **Choose 1 ounce of nuts or seeds over a "100-calorie pack."** These diet packages offer minimal calories but often no nutrition. Nuts, on the other hand, provide healthy fats and a little protein to help nourish your body with none of the added sugar. You can find convenient 1-ounce nut packs in your local grocery store or online.

5. **Choose low-sugar granola over traditional granola.** Typically, granola cereals and bars are high in sugar. Choose only those options with 6 grams of added sugar or less. Brands with low-sugar options include 18 Rabbits, Bear Naked Fit, and Purely Elizabeth. Just check the label because these brands also contain flavor combos that aren't so low in sugar. Want to make your own? Try this book's Maple-Date Granola (page 40).

TOOLS AT THE READY

You'll need some basic items to fill your healthy cooking tool kit.

ESSENTIAL EQUIPMENT

Having the right equipment will save you time and effort in your cooking. These are your absolute necessities for cooking at home:

→ Baking dishes: 9-by-9-inch and 9-by-12-inch baking dishes, 12-cup muffin tin, 5-by-9-inch loaf pan, large baking sheets
→ Blender
→ Can opener
→ Food processor
→ Meat thermometer
→ Mixing bowls of various sizes
→ Nonstick, ceramic, cast-iron, or stainless steel skillets: medium and large sizes (cast iron and stainless steel pans are best for cooking over high heat, so it's a good idea to have one of each type)
→ Pots and saucepans: 2-quart saucepan, medium soup pot, 8-quart stockpot
→ Rubber spatulas
→ Sharp chef's knife

NICE-TO-HAVE GADGETS

For developing your cooking skills or for added convenience, here is a list of gadgets you may want to consider adding to your kitchen:

→ Electric grill
→ High-speed blender
→ Immersion blender
→ Mini food processor/chopper
→ Multifunction food processor with various disks for grating and chopping
→ Rice maker with steamer attachment
→ Silicone microwave steamer basket with lid

MAKING HEALTHY EATING ACCESSIBLE

It's not easy to change poor eating habits like fast food binges, relying on processed foods, or opting for takeout instead of cooking for yourself. Common obstacles to healthy eating include difficult recipes, expensive or hard-to-find ingredients, and dishes that taste mediocre or bland. I've addressed these challenges with the following solutions to make healthy eating more accessible, inviting, and always tasty.

EASY-TO-FIND, BUDGET-FRIENDLY INGREDIENTS

This book primarily calls for affordable refrigerator and pantry staples that you can find easily at any grocery chain (or that you might already have in your kitchen). Any ingredient that may be a little pricier or harder to find is used across multiple recipes to make that investment worthwhile.

WEEKNIGHT RECIPES

Whether you are a busy homemaker, at work late into the evening, or simply overwhelmed with plenty to do, this book has got you covered. No one wants to finish their busy day only to spend hours in the kitchen. That's why **more than half of the recipes in this book take 30 minutes (or less) to make from start to finish.** These include breakfasts and a wide variety of entrées. Whether you are opting for a zesty bean dish, a one-pot chicken meal, or a savory beef dish, you have plenty of recipes to choose from. For a list of these time-saving recipes, refer to the Quick and Easy Meal Plan (page 20). **If convenience is a priority, I highly recommend prepping larger batches of the staple sauces and dressings in chapter 10 to keep on hand for use throughout the week.**

FLAVORS FOR THE WHOLE FAMILY

Cooking healthy for yourself is one thing, but pleasing an entire family is quite another. That's why I've created crowd-pleasing recipes with flavors that suit a wide variety of eaters—think lightened versions of mac-n-cheese, spaghetti and meatballs, and stir-fry. The Meals for Families plan (page 28) is your go-to guide. These meals serve six to feed your entire family.

BEGINNER SKILL LEVEL

Creating healthy, tasty meals shouldn't require a chef's touch. You can prepare delicious, nutritious meals whether or not you've spent years in the kitchen. The recipes in this book are practical and beginner-friendly, with the most basic cooking skills in mind. For example, you'll notice that many recipes call for using the microwave to steam vegetables. You'll also regularly see frozen ingredients, such as bell peppers and brown rice, which are pre-prepped to cut your cook time down and make meal times that much easier. The Quick and Easy Meal Plan (page 20) provides easy, accessible recipes that are ideal for new cooks, with the bonus that they don't take long to prepare.

MEAL PLANS

Having a meal plan will set you up for success—it's a no-brainer way to transition to healthier eating and may be a tool you keep around for the long haul. Meal plans take the guesswork out of choosing your meals, which means you won't have the stress of creating dishes on the fly. Each meal plan also includes a handy grocery list, so you buy only what you need to save time and prevent waste.

NUTRITION INFORMATION

Nutrition information is provided for every recipe in this book. This will help you gauge the nutritional balance of each meal. However, although it's wise to get plenty of protein and fiber and keep your caloric intake within reason, you don't have to be obsessed with the numbers. Rest assured that all the recipes are designed to fit within the guidelines of a balanced plate.

READING THE RECIPE LABELS

The last section covered the many tools this book offers to make healthy eating both attainable and accessible. You can navigate those tools using the labels provided with each recipe, choosing those that best fit your lifestyle needs. You can refer to the index at the back of the book to easily find recipes by label.

CONVENIENCE LABELS

From quick and easy to waste-free, you can choose the option that suits your cooking style:

30-Minute Meal: From start to finish, these meals will be done in half an hour or less. This includes both your prep and cook time.

One Pot/Pan: You need just one cooking vessel (e.g., a pot, pan, or oven-safe dish) for these dishes, which saves on cleanup time and keeps cooking simple.

Leftover-Friendly: You won't have to worry about flavors going awry or texture degrading with these dishes that store well in the refrigerator or freezer. In some cases, the dishes taste even better the next day.

DIETARY LABELS

The following labels pertain to those healthy eaters who must follow a special diet, whether you are sensitive to gluten, have nut allergies, or choose to follow a meat-free lifestyle:

→ **Gluten-free***
→ **Nut-free**
→ **Vegan**
→ **Vegetarian**

*Always check ingredient packaging for gluten-free labeling (in order to ensure that foods, especially oats, were processed in a completely gluten-free facility).

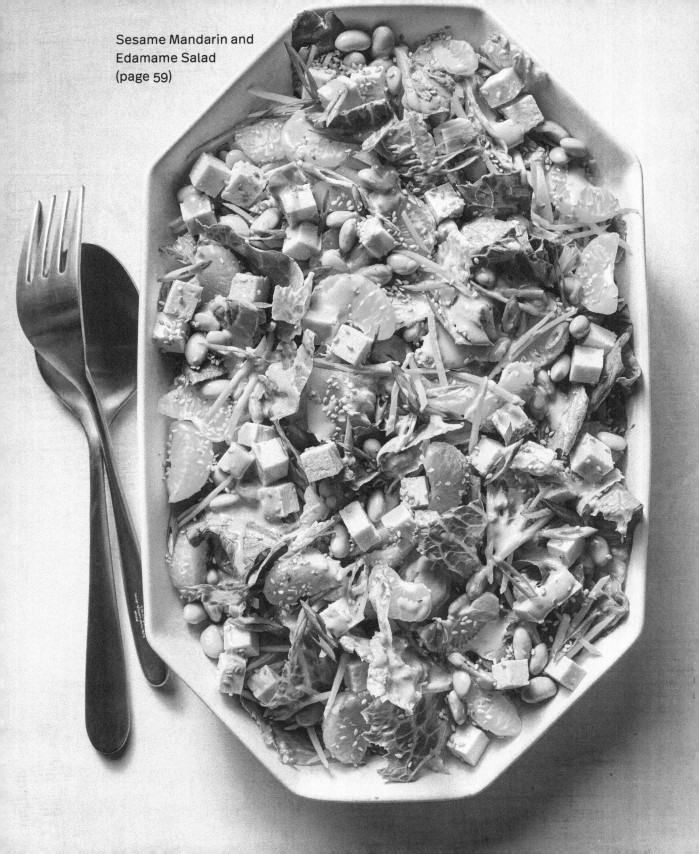

Sesame Mandarin and
Edamame Salad
(page 59)

CHAPTER 2

HEALTHY MEAL PLANS

When your diet is healthy, delicious, and convenient, it's easy to stick to. That's why meal plans are so effective; not feeling stressed about what to eat means you'll be less likely to make unhealthy choices for the sake of ease.

As the name implies, meal plans do require a bit of forethought, but that little bit of prep work ahead of time will save you hours in the kitchen come meal time. In addition to the meals suggested in the following plans, you'll get snack options for the week, tips for prepping ahead, and a detailed shopping list for each. Choose the plan that suits you best.

QUICK AND EASY MEAL PLAN

Short on time or new to cooking? The recipes in this plan were chosen because of their quick cook times and beginner skill levels. They are quick meals with minimal cooking know-how required.

WEEKLY MEAL PREP

Part of meal planning is prepping ahead. Choose a day and time when you can prepare some of the week's recipe elements to make assembling your meals even quicker. Here are some recipes and staples you should make in advance:

Dressings: Because both the Sesame Dressing (page 193) and Creamy Cilantro Dressing (page 194) are featured in a variety of dishes in this meal plan, you should prepare both of these the day before you start the plan. They will keep in airtight containers in the refrigerator for up to a week.

Banana-Nut Overnight Oats: The recipe is really quite simple. Just remember to check which days in the meal plan you'll be eating it so you can soak the oats the night before. Or prepare as many servings as you'll need for the entire week at once. They will last in individual airtight containers in the refrigerator for up to 5 days.

Strawberry-Spinach Salad with Lemon-Basil Vinaigrette: Prepare the Lemon-Basil Vinaigrette (page 192) ahead of time, and only dress the portion of salad you will eat when you serve it. Store leftover salad and dressing in separate airtight containers so the greens don't wilt.

Fiesta Chicken Macro Bowls: Chop the chicken into 1-inch chunks and prepare the DIY Taco Seasoning (page 198) the night before. Refrigerate the chicken in an airtight container until ready to use.

One-Pot Taco Shrimp: Defrost the shrimp in the refrigerator the night before to save time. You will have DIY Taco Seasoning (page 198) already prepared since it is used in a recipe earlier in the week.

Avocado tip: Unripe, hard avocados can be stored under bananas to speed ripening. Keep an eye on them daily. Store ripe avocados in the refrigerator if not using immediately.

	BREAKFAST	LUNCH	DINNER
SUNDAY	Pear, Spinach, and Ricotta Omelet (page 38)	Chickpea, Lentil, and Avocado Sandwiches (page 63)	Pineapple Chicken (page 126)
MONDAY	Banana-Nut Overnight Oats (page 36)	Strawberry-Spinach Salad with Lemon-Basil Vinaigrette (page 61) *(Can replace tofu with leftover Pineapple Chicken)*	Turkey Burgers with Creamy Cilantro Dressing (page 140)
TUESDAY	Cinnamon Oat and Pear Smoothie (page 46)	Leftover Turkey Burgers with Creamy Cilantro Dressing	Sesame Mandarin and Edamame Salad (page 59)
WEDNESDAY	Leftover Banana-Nut Overnight Oats	Leftover Strawberry-Spinach Salad with Lemon-Basil Vinaigrette	Fiesta Chicken Macro Bowls (page 124)
THURSDAY	Cinnamon Oat and Pear Smoothie (page 46)	Leftover Fiesta Chicken Macro Bowls	Ginger-Soy Noodle Bowls (page 82)
FRIDAY	Blueberry-Basil Avocado Toasts (page 34)	Leftover Ginger-Soy Noodle Bowls	One-Pot Taco Shrimp (page 99)
SATURDAY	Banana-Nut Overnight Oats (page 36)	Leftover One-Pot Taco Shrimp	Foil-Wrapped Tuscan Haddock (page 107)

SHOPPING LIST

MEAT/FISH/POULTRY/VEGAN PROTEIN

Chicken, boneless, skinless breast (12 ounces)

Chicken, boneless, skinless thighs (1 pound)

Haddock, 2 (6-ounce) fillets

Shrimp, medium, peeled, deveined, tails removed, frozen peeled, deveined, tails-off (1 pound)

Tofu, sprouted, firm (24 ounces)

Turkey, ground (12 ounces)

PRODUCE

Avocados, medium (5)

Bananas, medium (6)

Basil, fresh (1 bunch)

Blueberries (1 pint)

Broccoli, florets (10 ounces)

Carrots, medium (4)

Cilantro, fresh (1 bunch)

Cucumber, medium (1)

Garlic (1 bulb)

Ginger root (3-inch root)

Kale (4 bunches/20 ounces)

Lemons (5)

Lettuce, romaine (2 heads)

Oranges, Mandarin (2)

Pears, medium (6)

Scallions (1 bunch)

Spinach, baby (20 ounces)

Strawberries (2 pints)

Zucchini, medium (1)

DAIRY/DAIRY ALTERNATIVES AND EGGS

Almond milk (1 quart)

Cheese, part-skim ricotta (8 ounces)

Eggs, medium (½ dozen)

Milk, 1 percent (1 pint)

Yogurt, low-fat plain Greek (17.6 ounces)

CONDIMENTS AND SEASONINGS

Cayenne pepper

Cinnamon, ground

Cornstarch

Cumin, ground

Garlic powder

Honey

Mustard, Dijon

Nonstick cooking spray

Oil, canola

Oil, olive

Oregano, dried

Sea salt

Sesame seeds, toasted

Soy sauce, low-sodium

Tuscan seasoning

Vinegar, apple cider

Worcestershire sauce, low-sodium

CANNED, JARRED, OR PACKAGED

Almonds, sliced (2 tablespoons)

Beans, black, low-sodium, 1 (14½-ounce) can

Bread, whole-grain (1 loaf)

Broth, chicken, low-sodium (16 ounces)

Chickpeas, 2 (14-ounce) cans

Couscous, dried (10 ounces)

Dates, small pitted (5 ounces)

Hamburger buns, whole-wheat (4)

Lentils, brown or green, dried (¼ cup)

Noodles, instant ramen, 2 (3-ounce) packages

Oats, rolled, certified gluten-free if needed (4½ cups)

Pineapple, canned (8 ounces)

Tahini or peanut butter, all-natural (11 ounces)

Walnut halves (1 cup)

FREEZER

Bell pepper strips, tricolor, 4 (10-ounce) bags

Corn, sweet, 1 (10-ounce) bag

Edamame, shelled, 1 (10-ounce) bag

Green beans, 1 (10-ounce) bag

Rice, brown, 4 (10-ounce) bags

MEALS FOR WEIGHT LOSS

These are some of the leanest, meanest meals that will satisfy you while keeping those calories in check. Along with hydration and plenty of exercise, this is a plan you can count on to meet your weight loss needs.

WEEKLY MEAL PREP

Dressings/Staples: These dressings/staples are used in several of this plan's recipes. It is best to prepare them in advance so you'll have them ready in your arsenal of ingredients. Refrigerated in an airtight container, they stay fresh for up to a week.

→ Turmeric-Tahini Dressing (page 195): 1 batch
→ 5-Ingredient Mirepoix (page 199): 2 batches
→ Sesame Dressing (page 193): 1 batch
→ Date-Sweetened Barbecue Sauce (page 191): 1 batch

Carrot-Ginger Soup: Chop the carrots and shallots and mince the ginger and garlic; refrigerate in two separate airtight containers until ready to prepare.

Veggie Meatloaf: Prepare two batches of the 5-Ingredient Mirepoix (page 199) since this ingredient will be used in more than one recipe in this plan.

Tabbouleh Salad with Farro: You will need two batches of Tabbouleh Salad with Farro (page 58). Cut the tomatoes in half and chop the parsley and scallions; refrigerate separately in airtight containers. You'll squeeze the lemon and chop the cucumber the day you intend to serve your first plating. Once you've assembled the salad, enjoy your first portion and refrigerate the leftovers for components in future dishes (they will keep for up to 4 days).

Steak Salad with Sesame Dressing: Cut the steak into small strips and refrigerate in an airtight container for up to 3 days.

Banana-Nut Overnight Oats: The recipe is really quite simple. Just remember to check what days it falls on in the meal plan so you can soak the oats the night before.

	BREAKFAST	LUNCH	DINNER
SUNDAY	Cinnamon Toast Oatmeal (page 35)	Carrot-Ginger Soup (page 55) *(Supplement with steamed green beans)*	Tahini Roasted Salmon with Warm Kale Salad (page 110)
MONDAY	Green-Powered Smoothie (page 42)	Veggie Meatloaf (page 86)	Stuffed Eggplant with Savory Vegan Cream (page 76)
TUESDAY	Cinnamon Toast Oatmeal (page 35)	Leftover Stuffed Eggplant with Savory Vegan Cream	Leftover Carrot-Ginger Soup *(Supplement with leftover Warm Kale Salad)*
WEDNESDAY	Green-Powered Smoothie (page 42)	Tabbouleh Salad with Farro (page 58)	Mediterranean Bowls (page 79)
THURSDAY	Carrot, Mango, and Citrus Smoothie (page 45)	Butternut Squash and Tomato Soup (page 52) *(Supplement with steamed green beans)*	Veggie Meatloaf (page 86)
FRIDAY	Banana-Nut Overnight Oats (page 36)	Hummus Tabbouleh Wraps (page 64)	Steak Salad with Sesame Dressing (page 169)
SATURDAY	Carrot, Mango, and Citrus Smoothie (page 45)	Leftover Steak Salad with Sesame Dressing	Dijon Roasted Chicken with Grits (page 132)

SHOPPING LIST

MEAT/FISH/POULTRY

Beef, flank steak (1 pound)

Chicken, boneless, skinless
breasts (1 pound)

Salmon, 2 (6-ounce) fillets

PRODUCE

Apples, green (2)

Bananas, medium (3)

Basil, fresh (2 bunches)

Carrots, medium (20)

Celery (1 bunch)

Cilantro, fresh (1 bunch)

Cucumber (3 large or 6 small)

Eggplant, medium (1)

Garlic (2 bulbs)

Ginger root (6-inch piece)

Green beans (1½ pounds)

Kale, lacinato (2 bunches)

Lemons (5)

Lettuce, romaine (2 heads)

Mushrooms, white (15)

Onions, medium, yellow (6)

Oranges, Mandarin (3)

Parsley, fresh (3 bunches)

Potatoes, russet, medium (6)

Scallions (4 bunches)

Shallots (2)

Squash, butternut, medium (1)

Thyme, fresh (1 bunch)

Tomatoes, cherry (2 pints)

Tomatoes, vine-ripe, small (4)

Tomatoes, vine-ripe, medium (4)

DAIRY/DAIRY ALTERNATIVES AND EGGS

Almond milk (1 quart)

Cheese, feta (5 ounces)

Cheese, parmesan, grated
(4 ounces)

Eggs, medium (½ dozen)

Half-and-half (1 pint)

Milk, 1 percent (1 quart)

Yogurt, low-fat plain Greek
(17.6 ounces)

CONDIMENTS AND SEASONINGS

Capers

Cinnamon, ground

Cornstarch

Cumin, ground

Garlic powder
Honey
Maple syrup
Mustard, Dijon

Nonstick cooking spray

Oil, canola

Oil, olive

Onion powder

Sea salt

Sesame seeds, toasted

Tomato paste

Turmeric

Vinegar, apple cider

Worcestershire sauce, low-sodium, vegan

CANNED, JARRED, OR PACKAGED

Bread crumbs, panko (8 ounces)

Broth, chicken, low-sodium (1 quart)

Broth, vegetable, low-sodium (1 quart)

Chickpeas, 2 (15-ounce) cans

Coconut water (32 ounces)

Dates, small pitted (8 ounces)

Farro (2 cups)

Flax meal (1 pound)

Grits, instant (12 ounces)

Hummus (20 ounces)

Lentils, brown, dried (2¾ cups)

Marinara sauce, low-sodium (16 ounces)

Oats, rolled, certified gluten-free if needed (5⅓ cups)

Olives, green (8)

Soup, cream of mushroom, low-sodium (10½ ounces)

Tahini (11 ounces)

Tortillas, whole-grain, 8-inch (4)

Walnuts, halves (½ cup)

FREEZER

Corn, sweet, 1 (10-ounce) bag

Edamame, shelled, 1 (10-ounce) bag

Green beans, 1 (10-ounce) bag

Mango, chunks, 1 (10-ounce) bag

Rice, wild (1 pound)

MEALS FOR FAMILIES

If you are feeding a family, you're likely catering to various taste preferences (and maybe even picky eaters). This plan has a variety of crowd-pleasing, flavorful recipes with larger yields that are meant to feed families of up to six (with adult-size portions). If you have an extra-large family, double the recipes for leftovers. We realize that some kids live off Rice Krispies for breakfast and PB&Js for lunch, but they may very well enjoy chicken sandwiches and some of the reheated leftovers the next day.

WEEKLY MEAL PREP

Part of meal planning is prepping ahead. Choose a day and time when you can prepare some of the week's recipe elements to make assembling the recipes even quicker. Or prep the evening before. Here are a few recipes you can get a head start on.

Teriyaki Pork Stir-Fry: Make the Date-Sweetened Teriyaki Sauce (page 190). Slice the carrots. Cut the pork chops into ½-inch dice. Refrigerate separately in airtight containers until ready to use.

Black Bean Fiesta Bowls: Make the DIY Taco Seasoning (page 198) and store in an airtight container in the pantry. You'll be using this seasoning in a couple of recipes here (and in several more throughout the book), so it won't hurt to double the recipe. Make the Creamy Cilantro Dressing (page 194); refrigerate in an airtight container.

One-Pot Chicken with Penne and Tomatoes: Mince the garlic, grate the parmesan (if not buying pre-grated) and chop the chicken into 1-inch pieces (I recommend prepping the chicken the evening prior, but you can prep it up to 2 days in advance). Refrigerate separately in airtight containers until ready to use.

Beef and Broccoli Stir-Fry: Dice the steak and refrigerate in an airtight container for up to 5 days. Whisk together the soy sauce, honey, garlic, ginger, and cornstarch. Refrigerate in an airtight container until ready to use. Some contents may settle, so whisk again before using.

	BREAKFAST	LUNCH	DINNER
SUNDAY	Apple Flapjacks (page 48)	Teriyaki Pork Stir-Fry (page 157)	Simple Baked Chicken with Potato and Green Bean Salad (page 130)
MONDAY	Mango Cream Smoothie (page 43) *(triple this recipe to serve 6)*	Chicken, Lettuce, and Tomato Sandwiches with Creamy Cilantro Dressing (page 65) *(using the leftover Simple Baked Chicken)*	Leftover Teriyaki Pork Stir-Fry
TUESDAY	Cinnamon Toast Oatmeal (page 35)	Black Bean Fiesta Bowls (page 80)	One-Pot Chicken with Penne and Tomatoes (page 138)
WEDNESDAY	Tamale-Style Grits and Eggs (page 37)	Leftover One-Pot Chicken with Penne and Tomatoes	Beef and Broccoli Stir-Fry (page 166)
THURSDAY	Mango Cream Smoothie (page 43) *(triple this recipe to serve 6)*	Leftover Beef and Broccoli Stir-Fry	Chicken Parmesan (page 136)
FRIDAY	Blueberry-Basil Avocado Toasts (page 34)	Leftover Chicken Parmesan	Mexican-Inspired Tilapia with Bell Peppers and Kale (page 106)
SATURDAY	Cinnamon Toast Oatmeal (page 35)	Leftover Mexican-Inspired Tilapia with Bell Peppers and Kale	Stuffed Bell Peppers (page 160)

SHOPPING LIST

MEAT/FISH/POULTRY

Beef, flank steak (1½ pounds)

Beef, ground, 80 percent lean
(12 ounces)

Chicken, boneless, skinless
breasts (5¾ pounds/23 breasts)

Pork, 6 (4-ounce) boneless chops

Tilapia, 6 (4-ounce) fillets

PRODUCE

Apples, Fuji (4)

Avocados, medium (2)

Bananas, medium (6)

Basil, fresh (1 bunch)

Bell peppers, medium (6)

Blueberries (1 pint)

Broccoli, florets, small
(2¾ pounds)

Carrots (10 ounces)

Cilantro (1 bunch)

Garlic (2 bulbs)

Ginger root (6-inch root)

Kale (2 bunches)

Lemons (2)

Lettuce, romaine (2 heads)

Onions, yellow (3)

Potatoes, red, medium (5)

Scallions (1 bunch)

Spinach, baby (25 ounces)

Tomatoes, vine-ripe, medium (3)

DAIRY/DAIRY ALTERNATIVES AND EGGS

Cheese, parmesan, grated
(8 ounces)

Eggs, medium (1 dozen)

Milk, 1 percent (½ gallon)

Oat milk (1 quart)

Yogurt, low-fat plain Greek
(17.6 ounces)

CONDIMENTS AND SEASONINGS

Cayenne pepper

Cinnamon, ground

Cornstarch

Cumin, ground

Garlic powder

Honey

Italian seasoning

Lemon pepper seasoning

Maple syrup

Mustard, Dijon

Nonstick cooking spray

Oil, canola

Oil, olive

Oregano, dried

Sea salt

Soy sauce, low-sodium

Tomato paste

Vinegar, apple cider

CANNED, JARRED, OR PACKAGED

Almonds, raw, unsalted (½ cup)

Almonds, sliced (½ cup)

Applesauce, unsweetened
(23 ounces)

Baking soda (16 ounces)

Beans, black, 2 (15-ounce) cans

Bread, whole-grain (1 loaf)

Bread crumbs, panko (8 ounces)

Cashews, raw, unsalted (1½ cups)

Chocolate chips (8 ounces)

Coconut, flakes, unsweetened
(8 ounces)

Coconut, shredded, unsweetened
(12 ounces)

Dates, small pitted (12 ounces)

Flax meal (1 pound)

Flour, all-purpose (2 pounds)

Grits, corn (24 ounces)

Grits, instant yellow (18 ounces)

Hummus (10 ounces)

Marinara sauce, low-sodium
(48 ounces)

Oats, rolled (2 pounds)

Pasta, penne (12 ounces)

Peanut butter, all-natural
(16 ounces)

FREEZER

Bell pepper strips, tricolor,
4 (10-ounce) bags

Corn, sweet, 1 (14-ounce) bag

Green beans, 3 (10-ounce) bags

Mango, chunks, 1 (10-ounce) bag

Rice, brown, 4 (10-ounce) bags

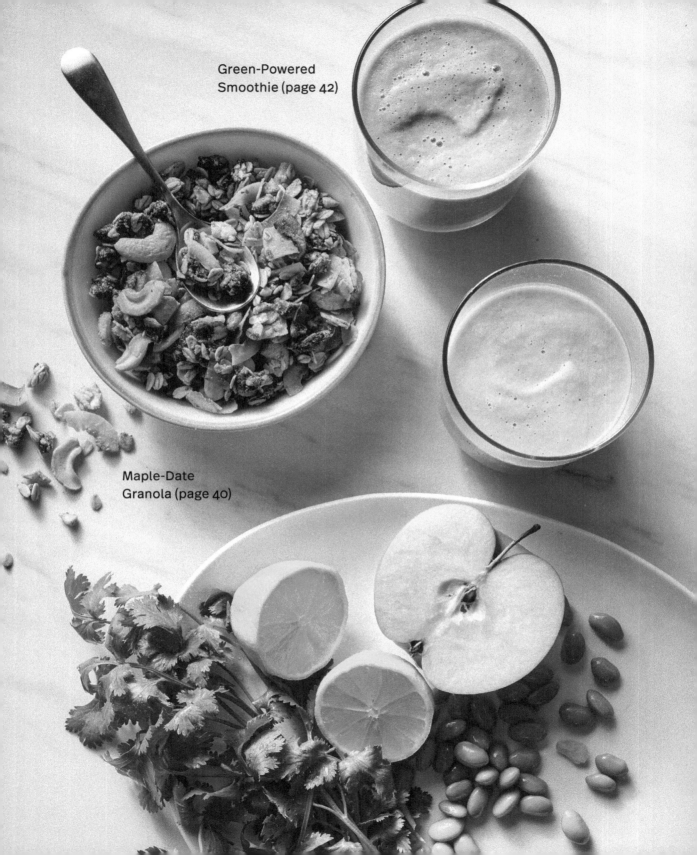

Green-Powered
Smoothie (page 42)

Maple-Date
Granola (page 40)

CHAPTER 3

BREAKFASTS AND SMOOTHIES

Blueberry-Basil Avocado Toasts **34**

Cinnamon Toast Oatmeal **35**

Banana-Nut Overnight Oats **36**

Tamale-Style Grits and Eggs **37**

Pear, Spinach, and Ricotta Omelet **38**

Maple-Date Granola **40**

Strawberry-Basil Smoothie **41**

Green-Powered Smoothie **42**

Mango Cream Smoothie **43**

Blueberry-Peach Smoothie **44**

Carrot, Mango, and Citrus Smoothie **45**

Cinnamon Oat and Pear Smoothie **46**

Coconut-Mango Green Smoothie **47**

Apple Flapjacks **48**

BLUEBERRY–BASIL AVOCADO TOASTS

SERVES 6 | PREP TIME: 5 MINUTES

30-MINUTE MEAL | VEGAN

Avocado toast is truly one of the best things ever—and so easy to make. Whether you choose to smash the avocado or arrange it in thin slices, it's a creamy base for a wide variety of options. This recipe is on the sweeter side, with fresh blueberries forming an inspired pair with the avocado. Garnished with fresh basil, it's a simple delight.

2 medium, ripe avocados, pitted, peeled, and sliced

6 whole-grain bread slices, toasted

1½ cups fresh blueberries

3 tablespoons julienned fresh basil leaves or baby spinach

PER SERVING (1 AVOCADO TOAST): Calories: 174; Fat: 8g; Carbohydrates: 22g; Protein: 5g; Fiber: 7g; Sodium: 85mg; Iron: 1mg

1. Divide the avocados evenly among the toast slices, mashing them into the toast if you like.

2. Top each slice with an equal amount of blueberries (you can crush some for ease of eating and variety in texture).

3. Garnish with the basil and serve.

TECHNICAL TIP: To create thin ribbons of basil, roll 6 to 8 leaves into a cigar shape with the smallest leaves in the center and the larger ones on the outside. Then, slice from end to end to form thin slices. This is called a chiffonade cut.

CINNAMON TOAST OATMEAL

SERVES 6 | PREP TIME: 5 MINUTES **| COOK TIME:** 10 MINUTES

30-MINUTE MEAL | GLUTEN-FREE | LEFTOVER-FRIENDLY | NUT-FREE | VEGETARIAN

A simple oatmeal can be so nourishing and just a touch of sweetness is all it needs to be delicious. This cinnamon toast oatmeal gets its name by mimicking the classic cinnamon-sugar flavor combo. The flax meal provides a granular texture similar to sugar but is much more nutritious with heart-healthy omega-3s and dietary fiber.

1½ cups low-fat
  (1 percent) milk

1½ cups water

2 cups rolled oats (certified
  gluten-free if needed)

6 small, pitted
  dates, chopped

6 teaspoons maple
  syrup, divided

2 teaspoons ground
  cinnamon

2 tablespoons flax meal

PER SERVING (⅔ CUP):
Calories: 269; Fat: 5g;
Carbohydrates: 50g; Protein:
10g; Fiber: 7g; Sodium: 49mg;
Iron: 2mg

1. In a medium pot, combine the milk, water, and oats. Bring to a boil over medium-high heat.

2. Reduce the heat to medium. Add the dates and 4 teaspoons of maple syrup. Simmer for 5 minutes or until thickened. Remove from the heat. Cover the pot.

3. To make the topping, in a small bowl, combine the remaining 2 teaspoons of maple syrup, the cinnamon, and flax meal.

4. When ready to serve, divide the oatmeal among 6 bowls. Sprinkle equal amounts of the topping over each.

BANANA-NUT OVERNIGHT OATS

SERVES 4 | PREP TIME: 5 MINUTES, PLUS 8 HOURS TO CHILL

GLUTEN-FREE | VEGAN

Prep your breakfast ahead easily and conveniently with these overnight oats. Just assemble, seal, and refrigerate. You'll wake up to perfectly portioned oatmeal that you can eat right out of the jar—it's delicious served cold.

1⅓ cups rolled oats (certified gluten-free if needed)

¼ cup chopped walnuts

8 small, pitted dates, chopped

2 medium bananas, sliced

2 cups unsweetened almond milk

PER SERVING (1 CUP):
Calories: 253; Fat: 1g; Carbohydrates: 45g; Protein: 6g; Fiber: 6g; Sodium: 89mg; Iron: 2mg

1. Fill 4 small sealable jars with ⅓ cup oats each.
2. Equally distribute the walnuts, dates, and bananas among the jars.
3. Pour ½ cup of almond milk into each jar.
4. Tightly seal the jars and shake to incorporate. Refrigerate for 8 hours or overnight. Serve cold, or warm in the microwave before enjoying.

SUBSTITUTION TIP: You can replace the almond milk with low-fat dairy milk (1 percent). It will no longer be a vegan recipe, but you'll get some additional protein.

TAMALE-STYLE GRITS AND EGGS

SERVES 6 | PREP TIME: 5 MINUTES **| COOK TIME:** 15 MINUTES

30-MINUTE MEAL | ONE POT/PAN | LEFTOVER-FRIENDLY

GLUTEN-FREE | NUT-FREE | VEGETARIAN

This deconstructed tamale uses corn grits and frozen corn in its base and tomato paste and taco seasoning for those Mexican-inspired flavors. You can always bump up the heat in this brunch-worthy option by drizzling on some hot sauce. Leftovers can be placed in a tightly sealed container and refrigerated for up to 4 days.

1 cup plus 2 tablespoons corn grits

½ cup frozen sweet corn

1½ cups low-fat (1 percent) milk

¼ teaspoon sea salt

6 medium eggs

6 tablespoons tomato paste

1½ teaspoons DIY Taco Seasoning (page 198)

6 cups loosely packed baby spinach or arugula

Sriracha sauce, for serving (optional)

PER SERVING (⅙ OF THE RECIPE): Calories: 182; Fat: 6g; Carbohydrates: 23g; Protein: 12g; Fiber: 3g; Sodium: 510mg; Iron: 5mg

1. In a large skillet, combine the grits, corn, milk, and salt. Heat over medium heat for about 4 minutes, or until the mixture begins to boil.

2. Reduce the heat to medium-low. Simmer for 3 to 4 minutes, or until the grits start to thicken.

3. Make 6 wells in the grits mixture and crack an egg into each.

4. Using a tablespoon, dot the tomato paste around the eggs, but do not mix it in. Cover the skillet and cook for 3 to 5 minutes, or until the egg whites are firm but the yolks are still runny. Turn off the heat. If any egg whites haven't firmed yet, scoop grits over them and cover for 1 to 2 minutes, until they cook through.

5. Sprinkle in the DIY Taco Seasoning and gently swirl to incorporate without breaking the yolks.

6. Divide the spinach evenly among 6 bowls.

7. Top with the grits and 1 egg per bowl.

8. Drizzle Sriracha sauce on top (if using). Serve warm.

PEAR, SPINACH, AND RICOTTA OMELET

SERVES 4 | **PREP TIME:** 5 MINUTES | **COOK TIME:** 10 MINUTES
30-MINUTE MEAL | **GLUTEN-FREE** | **NUT-FREE** | **VEGETARIAN**

Omelets are a practical way to get some veggies into your morning meal, and this one has a bit of fruit, too. I recommend using a non-stick or ceramic pan for this recipe to make folding and transferring the egg mixture easy.

6 medium eggs

2 tablespoons low-fat (1 percent) milk

2 teaspoons olive oil

1 small pinch sea salt

½ cup part-skim ricotta cheese

2 medium pears, cored and sliced

4 cups baby spinach

PER SERVING (¼ OMELET):
Calories: 222; Fat: 12g; Carbohydrates: 17g; Protein: 13g; Fiber: 3g; Sodium: 165mg; Iron: 2mg

1. In a medium bowl, whisk together the eggs and milk until well blended.

2. Place a medium nonstick or ceramic skillet over medium heat and pour in the oil. Heat for 30 seconds or until it starts to sizzle.

3. Pour in the egg mixture and cook undisturbed for 1 minute. Using a spatula, pull the egg slightly away from the edges of the skillet, then tilt to let the runny egg fill the space and maintain full coverage of the bottom. Continue to cook for another 4 minutes or until the eggs have firmed.

4. In a small bowl, stir the salt into the cheese.

5. Using a teaspoon, add the cheese in small dollops evenly over the surface of the eggs, then top evenly with the pears.

6. Reduce the heat to low. Top with the spinach. Cover the skillet and cook for 2 to 3 minutes, or until the spinach has wilted.

7. Use the spatula to gently flip one side of the eggs over the other, folding them in half. Remove from the heat.

8. Transfer the omelet to a large plate or cutting board and cut into 4 equal triangles.

SUBSTITUTION TIP: To make this recipe dairy-free, swap out the milk for unsweetened plant-based milk (such as oat milk or soy milk) and replace the ricotta with avocado slices.

MAPLE-DATE GRANOLA

MAKES 1½ CUPS | PREP TIME: 10 MINUTES **| COOK TIME:** 30 MINUTES

VEGAN

Crunchy granola is a perfect accompaniment to parfaits and smoothie bowls. And it's a great snack on its own. My granola uses whole-food ingredients, such as prunes and dates, to hit the sweet spot, with just a touch of maple syrup to pull it all together.

5 prunes, chopped

5 small, pitted dates, chopped

3 tablespoons whole cashews

2 tablespoons maple syrup

1 teaspoon vegetable oil

⅛ teaspoon sea salt

1 tablespoon almond flour

¼ cup unsweetened coconut flakes

¾ cup rolled oats

Nonstick cooking spray, for coating

PER SERVING (¼ CUP):
Calories: 164; Fat: 6g; Carbohydrates: 27g; Protein: 3g; Fiber: 3g; Sodium: 62mg; Iron: 1mg

1. Preheat the oven to 350°F.
2. In a food processor, combine the prunes, dates, and cashews. Process for 20 to 30 seconds, or until coarsely chopped.
3. Scrape the fruit-and-nut mixture to a medium bowl. Stir in the maple syrup, oil, salt, almond flour, and coconut flakes. Pour in the oats and mix until well incorporated.
4. Spread the mixture evenly into a 9-inch square baking dish.
5. Spray a light coating of cooking spray on top of the mixture to promote browning.
6. Transfer the baking dish to the oven and bake for 15 minutes. Stir and return to the oven. Bake for another 10 to 15 minutes, or until the granola is golden. Remove from the oven. Let cool completely until crisp, about 15 minutes. Transfer to an airtight container and store at room temperature for up to 2 weeks.

INGREDIENT TIP: Soak your prunes the night before making this recipe to make them plump, juicy, and easier to incorporate. Simply put 5 prunes in ½ cup water in an airtight jar and refrigerate overnight.

STRAWBERRY-BASIL SMOOTHIE

SERVES 2 | **PREP TIME:** 5 MINUTES, PLUS AT LEAST 2 HOURS TO SOAK

GLUTEN-FREE | NUT-FREE | VEGAN

This refreshing beverage is similar to a granita, an icy Italian drink. Strawberries form the bulk of this recipe, providing plenty of vitamin C, and water-packed cucumber adds debloating, anti-inflammatory qualities. Use frozen strawberries or cucumbers (or just add a few cubes of ice) for more froth. Feeding your family? Double up the recipe, or make a second batch.

1 tablespoon chia seeds

3 tablespoons water

1 medium, ripe avocado, pitted and peeled

1¼ cups halved strawberries

½ small cucumber, sliced

4 small, pitted dates

2 medium, fresh basil leaves

½ cup unsweetened coconut water

1. In a sealable container, combine the chia seeds and water. Shake well. Refrigerate for 2 to 3 hours, or overnight, until gelled.

2. Put the avocado, chia gel, strawberries, cucumber, dates, basil, and coconut water in a blender. Process until well combined. Serve immediately.

INGREDIENT TIP: Chia is a nutrient-dense seed that can expand to 10 times its size or more when soaked. Using chia is a great way to thicken recipes and add some healthy fat and fiber.

PER SERVING (14 OUNCES): Calories: 238; Fat: 13g; Carbohydrates: 32g; Protein: 5g; Fiber: 11g; Sodium: 42mg; Iron: 2mg

GREEN-POWERED SMOOTHIE

SERVES 2 | PREP TIME: 10 MINUTES

30-MINUTE MEAL | ONE POT/PAN | GLUTEN-FREE | NUT-FREE | VEGAN

Green apple, cucumber, cilantro, and edamame add up to a whole lot of green goodness in this plant-powered smoothie. If you've got a handful of baby spinach, you can toss it in, too. Feeding your family? Double up the recipe, or make a second batch.

1 medium green apple, unpeeled, cored and chopped

½ cup sliced peeled cucumber

2 tablespoons coarsely chopped fresh cilantro

3 tablespoons freshly squeezed lemon juice

¼ cup shelled edamame (preferably frozen)

1 cup unsweetened coconut water

Put the apple, cucumber, cilantro, lemon juice, edamame, and coconut water in a blender. Process until well combined. Serve immediately.

INGREDIENT TIP: Edamame (young, immature green soybeans) add a bit of plant-based protein to this smoothie. You can find them conveniently shelled in the fresh or frozen section of your supermarket.

PER SERVING (8 OUNCES):
Calories: 104; Fat: 1g; Protein: 4g; Carbohydrates: 22g; Fiber: 5g; Sodium: 35mg; Iron: 0.8mg

MANGO CREAM SMOOTHIE

SERVES 2 | PREP TIME: 5 MINUTES, PLUS OVERNIGHT TO SOAK

GLUTEN-FREE | VEGAN

Mango gives this smoothie an orange blush. For best results, soak your cashews overnight. Unsoaked raw cashews will do in a pinch, but the smoothie won't be as thick and creamy. Feeding your family? Double up the recipe, or make a second batch.

½ cup raw, unsalted cashews

1 cup water

1 banana, sliced

⅔ cup frozen mango chunks

1 cup unsweetened oat milk

PER SERVING (8 OUNCES):
Calories: 242; Fat: 10g; Carbohydrates: 37g; Protein: 5g; Fiber: 4g; Sodium: 53mg; Iron: 2mg

1. In an airtight jar, combine the cashews and water. Refrigerate overnight, then rinse and drain.

2. Put the soaked cashews, banana, mango, and oat milk in a blender. Process until well combined. Serve immediately.

SUBSTITUTION TIP: Any plant-based milk will work in this recipe.

BLUEBERRY-PEACH SMOOTHIE

SERVES 2 | **PREP TIME:** 10 MINUTES, PLUS AT LEAST 2 HOURS TO SOAK

GLUTEN-FREE | **NUT-FREE** | **VEGAN**

This peach-sweetened smoothie has an edamame base for added protein. It packs in antioxidant-rich blueberries, dark leafy greens, and superfood chia seeds, which contain large amounts of anti-inflammatory omega-3 fatty acids. Feeding your family? Double up the recipe, or make a second batch.

1 tablespoon chia seeds

3 tablespoons water

½ cup shelled edamame (preferably frozen)

1 cup quartered peaches

¼ cup blueberries

1 cup baby spinach

Juice of ½ lime

1 cup unsweetened coconut water

PER SERVING (8 OUNCES):
Calories: 125; Fat: 3g; Carbohydrates: 21g; Protein: 6g; Fiber: 7g; Sodium: 50mg; Iron: 2mg

1. In a sealable container, combine the chia seeds and water. Shake well. Refrigerate for 2 to 3 hours, or overnight, until gelled.

2. Put the edamame, chia gel, peaches, blueberries, spinach, lime juice, and coconut water in a blender. Process until well combined. Serve immediately.

INGREDIENT TIP: If it's not peach season, canned peaches are okay to use; just be sure to drain and rinse them beforehand to remove the excess sugars. If you have water-packed peaches, even better.

CARROT, MANGO, AND CITRUS SMOOTHIE

SERVES 2 | PREP TIME: 10 MINUTES

30-MINUTE MEAL | ONE POT/PAN | GLUTEN-FREE | NUT-FREE | VEGAN

This refreshing smoothie has notes of citrus and ginger, giving it a tangy, zesty appeal. The turmeric adds anti-inflammatory compounds, although its earthy flavor is quite subtle in this light refresher. Feeding your family? Double up the recipe, or make a second batch.

½ medium banana, sliced

½ cup shredded carrots

½ cup frozen
   mango chunks

1 Mandarin orange, peeled

2 teaspoons finely grated
   fresh ginger

½ teaspoon turmeric

1¼ cups unsweetened
   coconut water

Put the banana, carrots, mango, Mandarin orange, ginger, turmeric, and coconut water in a blender. Process until well combined. Serve immediately.

VARIATION TIP: Divide equally into 2 airtight containers and freeze to make 2 low-calorie sorbet snacks.

PER SERVING (8 OUNCES):
Calories: 100; Fat: 1g;
Carbohydrates: 52g; Protein:
2g; Fiber: 4g; Sodium: 52mg;
Iron: 1mg

CINNAMON OAT AND PEAR SMOOTHIE

SERVES 2 | PREP TIME: 5 MINUTES

30-MINUTE MEAL | ONE POT/PAN | GLUTEN-FREE | NUT-FREE | VEGAN

The combination of cinnamon and pear is a subtle variation on the more classic apple-cinnamon pairing that's popular in instant oatmeal and pastries. But the nutritional benefit of this smoothie surpasses many of those highly processed breakfast options. Oats keep this smoothie grounded with their natural supply of B vitamins and dietary fiber. Feeding your family? Double up the recipe, or make a second batch.

1 medium banana, peeled

1 cup diced pear (2 medium pears)

¼ teaspoon ground cinnamon

½ cup rolled oats (certified gluten-free if needed)

1 cup water

PER SERVING (8 OUNCES):
Calories: 220; Fat: 2g; Carbohydrates: 51g; Protein: 4g; Fiber: 9g; Sodium: 8mg; Iron: 1mg

Put the banana, pear, cinnamon, oats, and water in a blender. Process until well combined. Serve immediately.

SUBSTITUTION TIP: For added protein, replace the water with low-fat milk or unsweetened soy milk.

INGREDIENT TIP: If it's not pear season, canned pears are okay to use; just be sure to drain and rinse them beforehand to remove the excess sugars. If you have water-packed pears, even better.

COCONUT–MANGO GREEN SMOOTHIE

SERVES 2 | **PREP TIME:** 5 MINUTES

30-MINUTE MEAL | **GLUTEN-FREE** | **NUT-FREE** | **VEGAN**

Coconut and mango add a tropical flair to this refreshing smoothie. Antioxidant-rich with fiber and essential nutrients like vitamin C and potassium, this recipe provides a winning combo for immunity, digestive support, and weight control. Feeding your family? Double up the recipe, or make a second batch.

1 tablespoon flax meal

2 tablespoons water

1 medium banana, peeled

¾ cup frozen
mango chunks

¼ cup unsweetened
coconut flakes

1 teaspoon all-natural
peanut butter

1 cup baby spinach

1 cup unsweetened
coconut milk

1. In a small bowl, soak the flax meal in the water for 5 to 10 minutes, or until gelled.
2. Put the banana, flax gel, mango, coconut flakes, peanut butter, spinach, and coconut milk in a blender. Process until well combined. Serve immediately.

VARIATION TIP: Swap out the coconut milk for soy or oat milk, or keep it tropical by using unsweetened coconut water instead.

PER SERVING (8 OUNCES):
Calories: 181; Fat: 6g; Carbohydrates: 32g; Protein: 3g; Fiber: 5g; Sodium: 27mg; Iron: 2mg

APPLE FLAPJACKS

SERVES 6 | **PREP TIME:** 5 MINUTES | **COOK TIME:** 15 MINUTES
30-MINUTE MEAL | **LEFTOVER-FRIENDLY** | **NUT-FREE** | **VEGETARIAN**

These pancakes have applesauce both in the batter and as a topping, blended with maple syrup to keep them rich in apple flavor but low in added sugars. Fresh chopped apples give the pancakes a little crunch, too. Dust these pancakes with cinnamon and serve with a dollop of Greek yogurt, if you like.

1½ cups all-purpose flour

1½ teaspoons baking soda

¼ teaspoon salt

1½ cups low-fat (1 percent) milk

2 medium eggs

1½ cups unsweetened applesauce, divided

4 tablespoons canola or sunflower oil, divided

3 tablespoons maple syrup

¼ teaspoon ground cinnamon

3 small Fuji apples, cored and chopped

PER SERVING (2 PANCAKES WITH MAPLE-APPLESAUCE TOPPING): Calories: 333; Fat: 12g; Carbohydrates: 51g; Protein: 7g; Fiber: 3g; Sodium: 364mg; Iron: 2mg

1. To make the batter, in a medium bowl, combine the flour, baking soda, and salt. Mix well.

2. Add the milk, eggs, and ⅓ cup of applesauce. Stir until thoroughly combined.

3. Place a medium nonstick or ceramic skillet over medium heat and pour in 1 tablespoon of oil. Heat for 30 seconds, or until a small bit of batter dropped into the oil actively sizzles.

4. Using a ⅓-cup measuring cup or a 3-ounce ice cream scoop, transfer the batter into the skillet, 2 pancakes at a time. Cook for 1 to 2 minutes, or until you see bubbles in the batter.

5. Flip each pancake and cook for another minute, or until firm and golden brown. Repeat with the remaining batter, using 1 tablespoon of oil per 2 pancakes, until the batter is gone.

6. In a microwave-safe bowl, combine the remaining applesauce, the maple syrup, and cinnamon. Cover and heat for 30 seconds.

7. Serve each pancake with 3 tablespoons of maple applesauce and 1 to 2 tablespoons of chopped apple. Refrigerate leftovers separately in tightly sealed containers for up to 3 days.

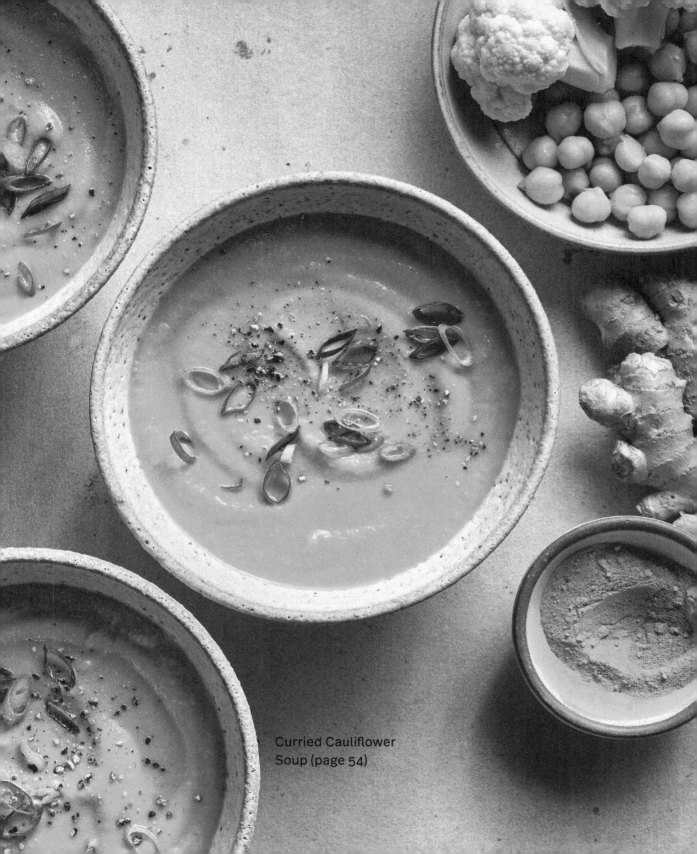

Curried Cauliflower
Soup (page 54)

CHAPTER 4

SOUPS, SALADS, AND SANDWICHES

Butternut Squash and Tomato Soup **52**

Lemony Lentil Soup **53**

Curried Cauliflower Soup **54**

Carrot-Ginger Soup **55**

Cream of Asparagus Soup **56**

Sesame Avocado Salad **57**

Tabbouleh Salad with Farro **58**

Sesame Mandarin and Edamame Salad **59**

Cucumber, Tomato, and Basil Salad **60**

Strawberry-Spinach Salad with Lemon-Basil Vinaigrette **61**

Apple and Walnut Salad over Greens **62**

Chickpea, Lentil, and Avocado Sandwiches **63**

Hummus Tabbouleh Wraps **64**

Chicken, Lettuce, and Tomato Sandwiches with Creamy Cilantro Dressing **65**

Smooth Zucchini Soup **66**

BUTTERNUT SQUASH AND TOMATO SOUP

SERVES 4 | **PREP TIME:** 15 MINUTES | **COOK TIME:** 45 MINUTES

LEFTOVER-FRIENDLY | **GLUTEN-FREE** | **NUT-FREE**

This herb-enhanced butternut squash soup gets its tang from roasted tomatoes, which are perfect alongside the creamy, mild sweetness of the squash. For a heartier flavor, swap out the chicken broth for low-sodium beef broth and add up to 2 teaspoons of low-sodium soy sauce.

2 cups chopped butternut squash

4 medium vine-ripened tomatoes, quartered

2 teaspoons olive oil, plus 1 tablespoon

Pinch sea salt

1 large yellow onion, chopped

1 to 2 tablespoons water

4 cups low-sodium chicken broth

2 teaspoons fresh thyme leaves

1 garlic clove, minced

½ cup plain low-fat Greek yogurt

PER SERVING (1½ CUPS):
Calories: 179; Fat: 7g; Protein: 7g; Carbohydrates: 24g; Fiber: 6g; Sodium: 221mg; Iron: 2mg

1. Preheat the oven to 375°F.
2. Put the squash and tomatoes on a baking sheet. Toss with 2 teaspoons of oil and the salt.
3. Transfer the baking sheet to the oven and bake for 40 minutes, or until the squash is soft and the tomatoes are puckered. Remove from the oven.
4. Meanwhile, in a medium soup pot, heat the remaining 1 tablespoon of oil over medium heat.
5. Add the onion and sauté for 5 to 7 minutes, or until soft and translucent.
6. Add the water as necessary to keep the onion from sticking.
7. Add the cooked squash and tomatoes to the pot along with the broth, thyme, and garlic. Cook for 5 to 7 minutes, or until the soup is warmed throughout. Remove from the heat.
8. Carefully transfer the soup to a blender. Process until smooth.
9. Serve the soup warm topped with the yogurt. Refrigerate any leftover soup in an airtight container for up to 4 days.

LEMONY LENTIL SOUP

SERVES 4 | PREP TIME: 10 MINUTES | **COOK TIME:** 35 TO 40 MINUTES

LEFTOVER-FRIENDLY | GLUTEN-FREE | NUT-FREE | VEGAN

This tangy, lemony lentil soup is partly pureed in order to get a creamy base while retaining some texture. It's a savory delight that pairs well with rice, tofu, and even eggplant, infusing those milder, starchy foods with its heady aromatics.

1 tablespoon olive oil

1 cup thinly sliced or chopped yellow onion

2 garlic cloves, minced

¼ teaspoon ground cumin

¼ teaspoon sea salt

2¼ cups water, divided

¼ cup freshly squeezed lemon juice

2 cups baby kale

1 medium carrot, chopped

½ cup dried brown lentils

PER SERVING (1 CUP):
Calories: 140; Fat: 4g; Protein: 12g; Carbohydrates: 21g; Fiber: 7g; Sodium: 167mg; Iron: 42mg

1. In a large skillet, heat the oil for 1 minute over medium heat.

2. Add the onion and cook for 10 minutes, or until completely softened.

3. Stir in the garlic, cumin, and salt. Cook for 30 seconds, or until fragrant.

4. Add ¾ cup of water, the lemon juice, kale, carrot, and lentils. Bring to a boil.

5. Reduce the heat to low. Cover the skillet and simmer for 20 minutes, or until the vegetables are tender.

6. Using an immersion blender, pulse the mixture halfway. Or transfer half the mixture to a food processor and process for about 1 minute, or until just creamy (some kale flecks should remain), then return the processed mixture to the skillet and stir until incorporated. Remove from the heat.

7. Serve the soup warm. Refrigerate leftover soup in an airtight container for up to 4 days.

INGREDIENT TIP: Kale is a dark, leafy green rich in vitamin K. It is usually necessary to massage raw mature kale to break down its tough fibers, but you don't have to worry about that with baby kale or when the kale is cooked.

CURRIED CAULIFLOWER SOUP

SERVES 4 | PREP TIME: 10 MINUTES | **COOK TIME:** 30 MINUTES

LEFTOVER-FRIENDLY | NUT-FREE | VEGAN

Reminiscent of Indian cuisine, this curried soup is full of mouth-warming spice. Chickpeas and cauliflower add a starchy appeal. Altogether, this anti-inflammatory dish is a well-balanced blend of robust flavor that is sure to delight with every spoonful.

1 tablespoon olive oil

1 cup chopped yellow onion

2 garlic cloves, minced

2 teaspoons minced fresh ginger

½ teaspoon ground cumin

½ teaspoon ground turmeric

1 tablespoon curry powder

3 tablespoons tomato paste

1 head cauliflower, green leaves removed, chopped

2 cups low-sodium vegetable broth

½ cup canned chickpeas, drained and rinsed

¼ cup chopped scallions, green parts only

PER SERVING (1½ CUPS):
Calories: 155; Fat: 5g; Protein: 7g; Carbohydrates: 42g; Fiber: 8g; Sodium: 442mg; Iron: 2mg

1. In a large skillet, heat the oil for 1 minute over medium heat.

2. Add the onion and cook for 5 minutes, or until softened.

3. Stir in the garlic, ginger, cumin, turmeric, and curry powder. Sauté for about 30 seconds, or until fragrant.

4. Stir in the tomato paste, cauliflower, broth, and chickpeas. Bring to a boil.

5. Reduce the heat to low. Cover the skillet and simmer for 20 minutes, or until the cauliflower is tender. Remove from the heat.

6. Transfer the soup to a blender. Process until smooth.

7. Garnish each serving with an equal amount of scallions. Serve warm. Refrigerate leftover soup in an airtight container for up to 4 days.

INGREDIENT TIP: Add a pinch or two of freshly ground black pepper to activate the turmeric's curcumin compounds for greater anti-inflammatory benefits.

CARROT-GINGER SOUP

SERVES 4 | **PREP TIME:** 10 MINUTES | **COOK TIME:** 40 TO 45 MINUTES

LEFTOVER-FRIENDLY | **GLUTEN-FREE** | **NUT-FREE** | **VEGETARIAN**

I love a creamy carrot soup. One of my favorite local restaurants makes it, but only on occasion, so getting it is often hit or miss. I created my own blend with a kick of ginger and savory seasonings to satisfy my frequent cravings for this nourishing soup.

2 tablespoons olive oil

⅛ teaspoon sea salt

¼ teaspoon ground cumin

1 tablespoon minced fresh ginger

½ cup chopped shallots

2 garlic cloves, minced

2 cups low-sodium vegetable broth

2 cups water

8 medium carrots, chopped

½ cup canned chickpeas, drained and rinsed

3 tablespoons half-and-half

PER SERVING (1½ CUPS):
Calories: 178; Fat: 9g; Protein: 4g; Carbohydrates: 23g; Fiber: 5g; Sodium: 542mg; Iron: 1mg

1. In a large stockpot, heat the oil over medium heat for about 1 minute, or until it starts to shimmer.

2. Add the salt, cumin, ginger, and shallots.

3. Reduce the heat to medium-low. Cook for about 8 minutes, or until the shallots are tender. Then add the garlic and cook for another 30 seconds until fragrant.

4. Add the broth, water, and carrots. Return the heat to medium. Bring to a boil.

5. Reduce the heat to medium-low again. Simmer for 30 minutes, or until the carrots are tender.

6. Add the chickpeas and half-and-half. Remove from the heat.

7. Transfer the soup to a blender. Process until smooth. Serve warm. Refrigerate leftover soup in an airtight container for up to 4 days.

VARIATION TIP: Add a squeeze of lemon and a bit of cilantro to brighten the dish before serving. Or if you've got sumac or grated lemon peel, you can use that instead of the lemon juice, which is an option for those who suffer from chronic acid reflux (or GERD).

CREAM OF ASPARAGUS SOUP

SERVES 4 | PREP TIME: 10 MINUTES **| COOK TIME:** 15 MINUTES

30-MINUTE MEAL | LEFTOVER-FRIENDLY | GLUTEN-FREE | NUT-FREE | VEGETARIAN

Creamy and green, this asparagus soup also features the umami of shiitake mushrooms and uses a special ingredient: edamame beans. Garlic and leek complete this warming bowl of comfort food goodness.

4 ounces trimmed asparagus, chopped

Nonstick cooking spray, for coating

Pinch salt

2 tablespoons canola oil

1 leek, white parts only, thoroughly rinsed and chopped

4 garlic cloves, minced

4 dried shiitake mushrooms

1 cup frozen shelled edamame, thawed

2 cups low-sodium vegetable broth

¼ cup half-and-half

PER SERVING (1½ CUPS):
Calories: 169; Fat: 10g; Protein: 7g; Carbohydrates: 14g; Fiber: 5g; Sodium: 354mg; Iron: 2mg

1. Preheat the oven to 400°F.
2. Spread the asparagus out on a baking sheet. Lightly coat with cooking spray. Sprinkle with the salt.
3. Transfer the baking sheet to the oven and roast for 15 minutes, or until the asparagus is tender. Remove from the oven.
4. Once the asparagus has roasted for about 10 minutes, place a medium pot over medium heat.
5. Pour in the oil and add the leek. Cook for 3 to 5 minutes, or until fragrant. Then add the garlic and cook for another 30 seconds until fragrant.
6. Add the mushrooms, edamame, broth, and half-and-half.
7. Reduce the heat to low. Add all but a few spears of the roasted asparagus to the pot; set aside the remaining asparagus for garnish. Remove from the heat.
8. Transfer the mixture to a blender. Process until smooth.
9. Garnish with the reserved asparagus and serve. Refrigerate leftover soup in an airtight container for up to 4 days.

SESAME AVOCADO SALAD

SERVES 6 | PREP TIME: 15 MINUTES

30-MINUTE MEAL | ONE POT/PAN | VEGETARIAN

Sesame adds a light, toasty crunch to the creaminess of avocado, a textural pairing that's oh-so-satisfying in this simple salad. It still packs in plenty of flavor, though, especially with the tangy kick of ginger pickled radish. (Remember that the pickled radishes take three days to cure, so prepare a batch ahead of time.)

8 cups chopped romaine lettuce

1 medium, ripe avocado, pitted, peeled, and chopped

1 cup Mandarin orange segments

¼ cup sliced Ginger Pickled Radish (page 200)

½ cup Sesame Dressing (page 193)

2 tablespoons sesame seeds, toasted

PER SERVING (1 CUP):
Calories: 141; Fat: 10g; Protein: 2g; Carbohydrates: 12g; Fiber: 5g; Sodium: 89mg; Iron: 1mg

1. Put the lettuce in a large salad bowl.
2. Reserving a few of each for garnish, add the avocado, Mandarin oranges, and pickled radish. Toss lightly to mix.
3. Add the dressing and toss again to coat.
4. Garnish with the remaining avocado, Mandarin orange segments, and radish, plus the sesame seeds. Serve immediately.

VARIATION TIP: Give this dish a more tropical feel by replacing the Mandarin oranges with an equal amount of chopped fresh mango.

TABBOULEH SALAD WITH FARRO

SERVES 4 | **PREP TIME:** 15 MINUTES | **COOK TIME:** 30 MINUTES

LEFTOVER-FRIENDLY | **NUT-FREE** | **VEGAN**

Tabbouleh is an herb-based chopped salad common in Middle Eastern cuisine. This recipe is a version that provides some heartier bits within the finely chopped basil and parsley. It also replaces the traditional bulgur wheat with farro, an ancient grain with a nutty flavor and a chewy texture.

1 cup farro

1½ cups minced fresh parsley

1 cup minced fresh basil leaves

1 cup chopped scallions, green parts only

1½ cups diced cucumber

2 cups halved cherry tomatoes

¼ cup freshly squeezed lemon juice

¼ cup olive oil

⅛ teaspoon sea salt

PER SERVING (1 CUP):
Calories: 202; Fat: 14g; Protein: 4g; Carbohydrates: 18g; Fiber: 4g; Sodium: 82mg; Iron: 3mg

1. In a medium pot, cook the farro according to the package instructions. Let cool for at least 20 minutes.
2. In a large bowl, combine the parsley, basil, scallions, cucumber, tomatoes, and cooled farro.
3. In a small bowl, whisk together the lemon juice, oil, and salt. Pour onto the salad and toss to coat evenly. Serve.

VARIATION TIP: You can add a couple ounces of firm tofu per serving to boost the protein content and make this salad a complete meal.

SESAME MANDARIN AND EDAMAME SALAD

SERVES 4 | PREP TIME: 15 MINUTES

30-MINUTE MEAL | ONE POT/PAN | VEGAN

With edamame and tofu, this Asian-inspired salad really packs in the protein. It also boasts a satisfying mix of texture and flavor thanks to a variety of crisp veggies, some citrus, and a light sesame crunch. If you're not a fan of tofu, add another cup of edamame.

4 cups chopped romaine lettuce

2 Mandarin oranges, separated into segments

1 cup shelled edamame

1 cup grated carrots

8 ounces firm, sprouted tofu, cubed

¼ cup Sesame Dressing (page 193)

2 scallions, green parts only, chopped

2 tablespoons toasted sesame seeds

PER SERVING (1 CUP):
Calories: 233; Fat: 14g; Protein: 12g; Carbohydrates: 18g; Fiber: 46g; Sodium: 155mg; Iron: 3mg

1. In a large salad bowl, combine the lettuce, Mandarin oranges, edamame, carrots and tofu.

2. Add the dressing, and toss to coat evenly.

3. Garnish with the scallions and sesame seeds. Serve.

INGREDIENT TIP: Traditional tofu is soft and will be too mushy for this salad unless you remove some water from it beforehand. To save on the pressing and draining time, buy firm tofu, which has less water and holds its shape. I recommend sprouted tofu for its nutritional qualities since it contains more protein and calcium than traditional tofu.

CUCUMBER, TOMATO, AND BASIL SALAD

SERVES 4 | PREP TIME: 15 MINUTES **| COOK TIME:** 20 MINUTES

GLUTEN-FREE | NUT-FREE | VEGAN

The simplicity of four common ingredients makes this refreshing salad an easy go-to. Lemon and simple seasoning add interest without overpowering the natural flavors of ripe tomatoes, crisp cucumber, and pungent, sweet basil.

1 cup quinoa

½ large cucumber, coarsely chopped

1 cup halved cherry tomatoes

¼ cup julienned fresh basil leaves

1 cup canned chickpeas, drained and rinsed

¼ cup freshly squeezed lemon juice

2 tablespoons olive oil

¼ teaspoon sea salt

¼ teaspoon freshly ground black pepper (optional)

PER SERVING (1 CUP):
Calories: 192; Fat: 9g; Protein: 6g; Carbohydrates: 24g; Fiber: 5g; Sodium: 97mg; Iron: 2mg

1. In a medium pot, cook the quinoa according to the package instructions. Transfer to a plate. Cool in the refrigerator for 3 to 5 minutes.

2. In a medium salad bowl, combine the cucumber, tomatoes, cooled quinoa, basil, and chickpeas.

3. In a small bowl, whisk together the lemon juice, oil, salt, and pepper (if using). Pour onto the salad, and lightly toss to coat evenly.

VARIATION TIP: This salad is equally brightened with 6 tablespoons Lemon-Basil Vinaigrette (page 192).

STRAWBERRY-SPINACH SALAD WITH LEMON-BASIL VINAIGRETTE

SERVES 6 | PREP TIME: 5 MINUTES **| COOK TIME:** 5 MINUTES

30-MINUTE MEAL | GLUTEN-FREE | VEGAN

What's more refreshing than strawberries in a salad? Toasted walnuts add a nice crunch, and with spinach as the salad base, you get plenty of iron and calcium. Lemon-basil vinaigrette is a complementary pairing, but this salad is versatile enough for you to choose your favorite dressing.

3 tablespoons
walnut halves

¼ cup Lemon-Basil
Vinaigrette (page 192)

6 cups baby spinach

2½ cups halved
strawberries

8 ounces firm, sprouted
tofu, cubed

PER SERVING (1 CUP):
Calories: 172; Fat: 11g;
Protein: 10g; Carbohydrates:
11g; Fiber: 4g; Sodium: 42mg;
Iron: 3mg

1. In a small skillet, toast the walnuts over medium heat, stirring occasionally, for 2 to 3 minutes, or until browned and fragrant. Remove from the heat.

2. In a large salad bowl, combine the vinaigrette, walnuts, spinach, strawberries, and tofu. Toss well. Serve.

SUBSTITUTION TIP: If you prefer animal protein, swap out the tofu for leftover cooked chicken or salmon.

APPLE AND WALNUT SALAD OVER GREENS

SERVES 4 | PREP TIME: 10 MINUTES

30-MINUTE MEAL | GLUTEN-FREE | VEGETARIAN

This dish can easily become a dessert or sweet snack if you simply omit the greens (although greens are always welcome in my book). But surprisingly, there are few added sugars—the salad is mostly wholesome whole foods. And you don't need much to make this one: just a few ingredients and a food processor or handheld food chopper.

2 large green apples, cored and coarsely chopped

½ cup walnut halves

8 small, pitted dates

4 cups chopped romaine lettuce

3 tablespoons freshly squeezed lemon juice, divided

Pinch sea salt

¼ cup plain low-fat Greek yogurt

2 tablespoons water

2 teaspoons honey

Pinch ground cinnamon, for garnish (optional)

1. Put the apples, walnuts, and dates in a food processor. Pulse a few times until the mixture is coarse and sticking together.

2. In a large bowl, combine the lettuce, 2 tablespoons of lemon juice, and the salt. Toss to coat evenly.

3. Divide the lettuce equally among serving bowls. Top with equal amounts of the apple mixture.

4. To make the dressing, in a small bowl, combine the yogurt, water, remaining 1 tablespoon of lemon juice, and the honey.

5. Drizzle the salad with the dressing.

6. Dust with cinnamon (if using).

INGREDIENT TIP: Walnuts are an excellent option for plant-based omega-3s—just 1 ounce of them provides up to 10 percent of your daily iron needs.

PER SERVING (⅓ CUP APPLE-WALNUT MIXTURE OVER 1 CUP GREENS): Calories: 197; Fat: 10g; Protein: 5g; Carbohydrates: 26g; Fiber: 5g; Sodium: 47mg; Iron: 1mg

CHICKPEA, LENTIL, AND AVOCADO SANDWICHES

SERVES 2 | PREP TIME: 5 MINUTES **| COOK TIME:** 15 MINUTES
30-MINUTE MEAL | NUT-FREE | VEGETARIAN

Despite being completely plant based, these simple sandwiches have plenty of protein, mainly from its legumes, which are super beneficial because they contain B vitamins and plenty of fiber, too. Season with some flavorful cilantro dressing for a tasty kick.

¼ cup brown or green lentils

¾ cup water

½ cup canned chickpeas, drained and rinsed

¼ cup Creamy Cilantro Dressing (page 194)

4 whole-grain bread slices, divided

8 crisp romaine lettuce leaves

1 medium, ripe avocado, pitted, peeled, and mashed

PER SERVING (1 SANDWICH):
Calories: 458; Fat: 18g; Carbohydrates: 58g; Protein: 20g; Fiber: 19g; Sodium: 480mg; Iron: 5mg

1. In a medium saucepan, combine the lentils and water. Bring to a boil over medium heat.
2. Reduce the heat to low. Cover the saucepan and simmer for 12 to 14 minutes, or until the lentils are tender. Remove from the heat. Drain any excess water.
3. In a small bowl, mash the lentils and chickpeas.
4. Mix in the dressing until well combined.
5. Pile the lentil-chickpea mixture on top of 2 bread slices.
6. Add the lettuce leaves.
7. Spread the avocado on the remaining 2 bread slices. Carefully stack on top of the lettuce.
8. Cut each sandwich in half and serve.

SUBSTITUTION TIP: If you're missing one of the legumes, you can easily swap out the chickpeas for lentils or vice versa.

HUMMUS TABBOULEH WRAPS

SERVES 4 | PREP TIME: 15 MINUTES

30-MINUTE MEAL | ONE POT/PAN | NUT-FREE | VEGAN

For this Middle Eastern–inspired sandwich, I chose some staples of the cuisine—chickpeas, tahini, and tangy tabbouleh. They're all wrapped up in a tortilla for a street-food feel.

1 cup hummus

4 (8-inch) whole-grain tortillas

1 cup Tabbouleh Salad with Farro (page 58)

1 cup chopped romaine lettuce

¼ cup Turmeric-Tahini Dressing (page 195)

PER SERVING (1 WRAP): Calories: 375; Fat: 17g; Carbohydrates: 45g; Protein: 14g; Fiber: 11g; Sodium: 588mg; Iron: 5mg

1. Spread ¼ cup of hummus over each tortilla.
2. Add ¼ cup of tabbouleh and ¼ cup of lettuce to each.
3. Roll the tortillas to form wraps.
4. Slice each in half and serve with a drizzle of dressing.

VARIATION TIP: If you've got a large, fresh collard green, you can use the leaves instead of tortillas to make the meal lower in carbohydrates.

CHICKEN, LETTUCE, AND TOMATO SANDWICHES WITH CREAMY CILANTRO DRESSING

SERVES 6 | **PREP TIME:** 5 MINUTES | **COOK TIME:** 25 MINUTES

30-MINUTE MEAL | **ONE POT/PAN** | **NUT-FREE**

The baked chicken in this sandwich is tender and juicy, thanks to a simple method of lightly coating with oil, adding a touch of sea salt, and sealing in aluminum foil to cook. The creamy cilantro dressing adds a nice tangy kick. Altogether, this sandwich is satisfying and tasty.

Nonstick cooking spray, for coating the baking dish

6 (4-ounce, ½-inch-thick) boneless, skinless chicken breasts

1½ tablespoons olive oil

¼ teaspoon sea salt

¼ cup plus 2 tablespoons hummus

12 whole-grain bread slices, divided

12 crisp romaine lettuce leaves

3 medium vine-ripened tomatoes, sliced

6 tablespoons Creamy Cilantro Dressing (page 194)

1. Preheat the oven to 425°F. Lightly coat a 9-by-13-inch baking dish with cooking spray.
2. Coat both sides of each chicken breast with the olive oil. Season with the salt.
3. Place the chicken in the prepared baking dish. Seal with aluminum foil.
4. Transfer the baking dish to the oven and bake for 20 to 25 minutes, or until the juices run clear. Remove from the oven. Let cool.
5. Spread the hummus on 6 bread slices.
6. Top each with 2 lettuce leaves, 1 chicken breast, and 2 tomato slices.
7. Drizzle each with 1 tablespoon of dressing.
8. Top each with the remaining 6 bread slices and serve.

INGREDIENT TIP: Hummus made from chickpeas and tahini is a great way to get in some vegetable protein and a little fiber. It also keeps this sandwich lighter in fats (swapping out traditional mayonnaise for this condiment).

PER SERVING (1 SANDWICH): Calories: 381; Fat: 13g; Carbohydrates: 22g; Protein: 43g; Fiber: 6g; Sodium: 392mg; Iron: 3mg

SMOOTH ZUCCHINI SOUP

SERVES 4 | PREP TIME: 10 MINUTES | **COOK TIME:** 25 MINUTES

LEFTOVER-FRIENDLY | NUT-FREE

This soup gets its creaminess from blending the broth with leek, zucchini, and lentils, the last of which contributes protein while thickening the soup. Greek yogurt adds a creamy garnish, which you can swirl in and enjoy as you sip the soup.

6 teaspoons olive oil, divided

1 large leek (white parts only, thoroughly rinsed) or medium yellow onion, sliced

2 garlic cloves, minced

⅛ teaspoon sea salt

1 tablespoon Italian seasoning

8 medium zucchini, peeled and coarsely chopped

2¼ cups low-sodium beef broth

1 cup arugula

¼ cup dried brown or green lentils

¾ cup water

½ cup plain low-fat Greek yogurt

PER SERVING (1½ CUPS):
Calories: 207; Fat: 9g; Protein: 13g; Carbohydrates: 23g; Fiber: 6g; Sodium: 356mg; Iron: 4mg

1. In a large skillet, heat 2 teaspoons of oil over medium heat for 1 minute.

2. Add the leek, garlic, salt, and Italian seasoning. Stir to incorporate and cook for about 7 minutes, or until the leek starts to soften.

3. Add the zucchini. Cover the skillet and cook for 12 minutes, or until the zucchini becomes soft.

4. Add the broth and arugula. Cover again and cook for about 2 minutes, or until the arugula has wilted. Remove from the heat.

5. While the soup is cooking, prepare the lentils. In a medium saucepan, combine the lentils and water. Bring to a boil over medium heat.

6. Reduce the heat to low. Cover the saucepan and simmer for 12 to 14 minutes, or until the lentils are tender. Remove from the heat. Drain any excess water.

7. Transfer the soup mixture to a blender. Add the lentils and process until fully pureed.

8. Divide the soup among 4 bowls. Garnish each with 2 tablespoons of yogurt.

9. Drizzle 1 teaspoon of oil into each bowl. Serve warm. Refrigerate leftover soup in an airtight container for up to 4 days.

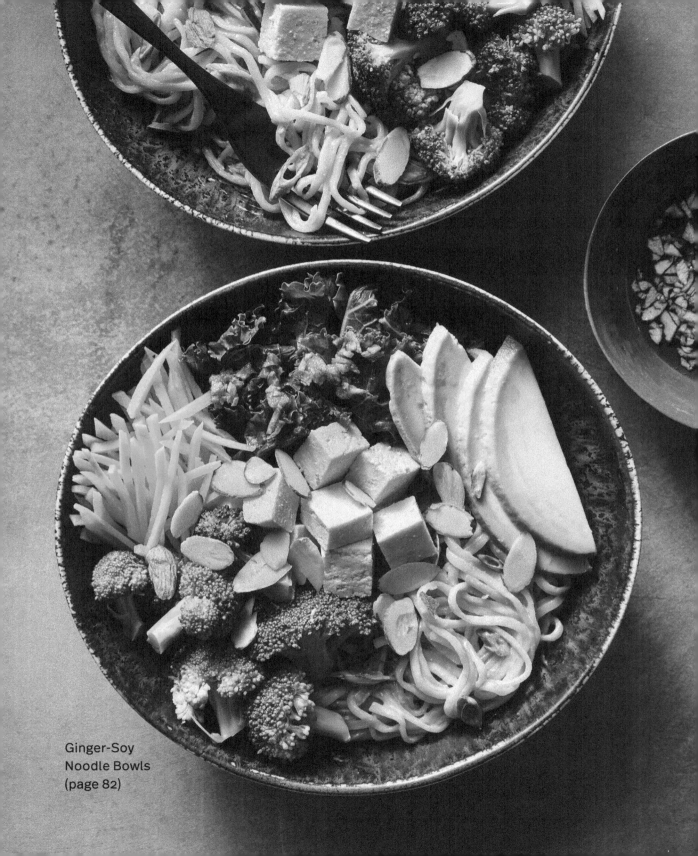

Ginger-Soy
Noodle Bowls
(page 82)

CHAPTER 5

VEGAN/VEGETARIAN

Lentil "Meat"balls with Basil and Parmesan **70**

Teriyaki Black Bean Burgers **72**

Teriyaki Veggie Stir Fry **74**

Sautéed Eggplant with Peppers and Onions **75**

Stuffed Eggplant with Savory Vegan Cream **76**

Chickpea, Kale, and Sweet Potato Bowls **78**

Mediterranean Bowls **79**

Black Bean Fiesta Bowls **80**

Quinoa Harvest Bowls **81**

Ginger-Soy Noodle Bowls **82**

Curried Lentil Stew **83**

Veggie Burger Parmesan **84**

Veggie Meatloaf **86**

Vegetarian Shepherd's Pie **88**

Roasted Veggie Mac-n-Cheese Au Gratin **90**

Spaghetti and Vegetarian "Meat"balls **92**

LENTIL "MEAT"BALLS WITH BASIL AND PARMESAN

SERVES 4 | **PREP TIME:** 10 MINUTES, PLUS 30 MINUTES TO CHILL |
COOK TIME: 35 TO 40 MINUTES

LEFTOVER-FRIENDLY | **NUT-FREE** | **VEGETARIAN**

You can cook the lentils from scratch as directed here, but this recipe is also a great way to use leftover cooked lentils when you want another option besides soup. The basil and parmesan pair well with the tomato-based ingredients for an Italian-inspired vegetarian dish. Don't skip the chilling step; it helps the mixture firm up for the best-texture "meat"balls.

Nonstick cooking spray, for coating

¾ cup dried brown lentils, rinsed

2½ cups water, divided

2 teaspoons olive oil

1 cup panko bread crumbs

1 tablespoon garlic powder

3 tablespoons finely chopped fresh basil leaves

½ cup grated parmesan cheese, divided

1 medium egg

¼ cup tomato paste

1 cup marinara sauce

2 cups frozen brown rice

2 cups fresh or frozen sliced carrots

1. Preheat the oven to 350°F. Line a rimmed baking sheet or a 9-by-13-inch baking dish with aluminum foil. Coat with cooking spray.

2. In a medium saucepan, combine the lentils and 2¼ cups of water. Bring to a boil over medium heat.

3. Reduce the heat to low. Cover the saucepan and simmer for 12 to 14 minutes, or until the lentils are tender. Remove from the heat. Drain any excess water.

4. To make the "meat"ball mixture, in a medium mixing bowl, combine the lentils, olive oil, bread crumbs, garlic powder, basil, ¼ cup of cheese, the egg, and tomato paste. Using a fork, mash until well combined. Cover and chill in the refrigerator for 30 minutes.

5. Scoop the batter into 1½-inch balls. Place on the prepared baking sheet.

6. Pour the marinara sauce evenly on top.

7. Transfer the baking sheet to the oven and bake for 20 minutes, or until the meatballs are firm and warmed throughout. Remove from the oven.

8. Garnish with the remaining ¼ cup of cheese.

9. Meanwhile, prepare the rice in the microwave according to the package instructions, usually about 3 minutes.

10. In a microwave-safe bowl, combine the carrots and remaining ¼ cup of water. Cover and microwave for 4 minutes, or until tender. Drain any excess water.

11. Serve the "meat"balls over the rice with the carrots on the side.

SUBSTITUTION TIP: To make this gluten-free, substitute 1 cup certified gluten-free oats for the bread crumbs. Grind them in a food processor beforehand for a finer texture.

PER SERVING (¼ OF THE RECIPE): Calories: 416; Fat: 10g; Carbohydrates: 66g; Protein: 18g; Fiber: 11g; Sodium: 561mg; Iron: 5mg

TERIYAKI BLACK BEAN BURGERS

SERVES 6 | **PREP TIME:** 10 MINUTES, PLUS 30 MINUTES TO CHILL | **COOK TIME:** 40 MINUTES

LEFTOVER-FRIENDLY | **NUT-FREE** | **VEGETARIAN**

Zesty and full of flavor, these burgers are a delicious way to get in plenty of fiber and plant-based protein. My date-sweetened teriyaki sauce gives it that extra kick of flavor to keep your mouth watering.

1 (14½-ounce) can low-sodium black beans, drained and rinsed

⅓ cup chopped yellow onions

2 garlic cloves, minced

¾ cup Date-Sweetened Teriyaki Sauce (page 190), divided

1¼ cups panko bread crumbs

1 medium egg

¼ cup tomato paste

¼ cup chopped scallions, plus 2 tablespoons, green parts only

5 tablespoons olive oil, divided

2 medium russet potatoes, scrubbed and cut into ½-inch wedges

¼ teaspoon sea salt, divided

4 cups romaine lettuce

2 cups shredded carrots

1. Preheat the oven to 425°F. Line a 9-by-13-inch baking dish with aluminum foil. Line a baking sheet with parchment paper.

2. In a food processor, combine the beans, onions, garlic, ½ cup of teriyaki sauce, the bread crumbs, egg, tomato paste, ¼ cup of scallions, and 1 tablespoon of oil. Process for about 1 minute until a thick paste forms. Transfer to a bowl.

3. Mold into 6 equal patties about 3 inches wide and ½-inch thick. Place in a single layer on a large plate. Cover and chill in the refrigerator for 30 minutes to firm.

4. Meanwhile, spread the potatoes into a single layer in the baking dish. Drizzle with 1 tablespoon of oil and ⅛ teaspoon of salt. Toss to coat.

5. Transfer the baking dish to the oven and bake for 30 minutes, or until the potatoes are tender and lightly browned.

6. In a large skillet, heat 2½ tablespoons of oil over medium-high heat for about 1 minute until shimmering.

7. Add the patties. Reduce the heat to medium. Cook for 3 to 5 minutes per side, or until lightly browned and crisp. Remove from the heat.

8. In a salad bowl, toss together the lettuce, carrots, remaining ⅛ teaspoon of salt, ½ tablespoon of oil, and 2 tablespoons of scallions.

9. Pour the remaining ¼ cup of teriyaki sauce equally onto each patty. Serve with the salad and potatoes on the side.

TECHNICAL TIP: To easily season potatoes, place them in a large airtight bag, add the oil and salt, and shake vigorously to fully coat.

PER SERVING (⅙ OF THE RECIPE): Calories: 343; Fat: 14g; Carbohydrates: 47g; Protein: 10g; Fiber: 9g; Sodium: 454mg; Iron: 3mg

TERIYAKI VEGGIE STIR-FRY

SERVES 4 | PREP TIME: 10 MINUTES | COOK TIME: 15 MINUTES

30-MINUTE MEAL | ONE-POT/PAN | NUT-FREE | VEGAN

A stir-fry is one of my favorite one-pot meals because I get to use a variety of colorful vegetables. For this recipe, I chose broccoli, bell pepper, and carrots, with mushrooms for a "meaty" addition. My date-sweetened teriyaki sauce infuses the veggies with its strong flavor and together they are lovely served over rice.

2 cups frozen wild rice or brown rice

1 tablespoon canola or sunflower oil

1 cup sliced mushrooms

⅛ teaspoon sea salt

1 cup frozen tricolor bell pepper strips

1 cup frozen broccoli florets

¾ cup shredded carrots

¼ cup Date-Sweetened Teriyaki Sauce (page 190)

1 pound firm tofu, cubed

PER SERVING (¼ OF THE RECIPE): Calories: 280; Fat: 12g; Carbohydrates: 27g; Protein: 19g; Fiber: 4g; Sodium: 293mg; Iron: 4mg

1. Prepare the rice in the microwave according to the package instructions, usually about 3 minutes.

2. Meanwhile, in a large high-sided skillet or wok, heat the oil over medium heat for 1 minute, or until shimmering.

3. Add the mushrooms. Sprinkle with the salt. Sauté for 5 minutes, or until the mushrooms begin to soften.

4. Add the bell pepper, broccoli, and carrots. Cook for 7 minutes, or until the veggies have defrosted and warmed through.

5. Stir in the teriyaki sauce and fold in the tofu. Remove from the heat. Serve over the rice.

SUBSTITUTION TIP: Swap out the tofu for 6 scrambled eggs if you wish.

SAUTÉED EGGPLANT WITH PEPPERS AND ONIONS

SERVES 4 | PREP TIME: 10 MINUTES | **COOK TIME:** 35 MINUTES

LEFTOVER-FRIENDLY | GLUTEN-FREE | NUT-FREE | VEGAN

I love making sautéed eggplant. It requires so little effort and such little prep (no marinating time necessary). This dish uses plenty of other vegetables, too, to keep things colorful and nutrient dense.

2 tablespoons olive oil

1 cup chopped yellow onion

⅛ teaspoon sea salt

1 tablespoon DIY Taco Seasoning (page 198)

1 teaspoon garlic powder

1 medium eggplant, cut into 1-inch dice

1 cup frozen tricolor bell pepper strips

4 cups baby spinach

2 cups Sweet Potato Medallions (page 203)

PER SERVING (¼ OF THE RECIPE): Calories: 235; Fat: 9g; Carbohydrates: 34g; Protein: 11g; Fiber: 13g; Sodium: 665mg; Iron: 9mg

1. In a large sauté pan, heat the oil over medium heat for 30 seconds.

2. Add the onion, salt, taco seasoning, and garlic powder. Sauté for 7 minutes, or until translucent.

3. Add the eggplant and bell pepper, tossing well. Cook for 25 minutes, or until the vegetables have softened. If they begin to stick or burn, reduce the heat, and add 1 to 2 tablespoons of water. Remove from the heat.

4. Fill a medium pot with a few inches of water and set a steamer basket inside it. Bring to a boil over medium heat.

5. Put the spinach in the steamer. Cover the pot and cook for about 3 minutes, or until just wilted. Remove from the heat.

6. Serve the vegetable mixture over the spinach with the sweet potatoes on the side.

TECHNICAL TIP: Use fresh eggplant, because the older it gets, the more bitter it will be. If you choose, you can salt the eggplant over a colander and let it drain for an hour to remove bitterness. Rinse before using.

STUFFED EGGPLANT WITH SAVORY VEGAN CREAM

SERVES 4 | PREP TIME: 15 MINUTES **| COOK TIME:** 30 MINUTES

LEFTOVER-FRIENDLY | GLUTEN-FREE | NUT-FREE | VEGAN

Melt-in-your-mouth eggplant pairs nicely with the colorful vegetable mélange in this satisfying meal. And best of all, you get to eat the bowl, since the eggplant is both the star and the serving vessel.

Nonstick cooking spray, for coating

1 medium eggplant

2 tablespoons olive oil, divided

⅛ teaspoon sea salt

¾ cup dried brown lentils, rinsed

2¼ cups water

2 garlic cloves, minced

1 recipe 5-Ingredient Mirepoix (page 199)

1 pound frozen wild rice or brown rice

¼ cup Turmeric-Tahini Dressing (page 195)

2 teaspoons toasted sesame seeds

PER SERVING (½ STUFFED EGGPLANT): Calories: 273; Fat: 11g; Carbohydrates: 38g; Protein: 10g; Fiber: 10g; Sodium: 193mg; Iron: 3mg

1. Preheat the oven to 425°F. Line a rimmed baking sheet or a 9-by-13-inch baking dish with aluminum foil. Coat with cooking spray.

2. Slice the eggplant in half lengthwise. Then, using a paring knife, hollow out the center, leaving a ¼-inch perimeter of flesh. Place the halves, cut-side up, on the prepared baking sheet. Drizzle with 1 tablespoon of olive oil. Sprinkle with the salt.

3. Turn the eggplant cut-side down.

4. Transfer the baking sheet to the oven and bake for about 30 minutes, or until the flesh becomes soft and the skin starts to pucker. Remove from the oven.

5. Meanwhile, prepare the lentils. In a medium saucepan, combine the lentils and water. Bring to a boil over medium heat.

6. Reduce the heat to low. Cover the saucepan and simmer for 12 to 14 minutes, or until the lentils are tender. Remove from the heat. Drain any excess water.

7. In a frying pan, heat the remaining 1 tablespoon of oil over medium-low heat for about 1 minute, or until shimmering.

8. Add the garlic, mirepoix, and cooked lentils. Cook, stirring occasionally, for about 5 minutes, or until the garlic is fragrant. Cover the pan and remove from the heat.

9. Prepare the rice in the microwave according to the package instructions, usually about 3 minutes.

10. Once the eggplant is done, fill each eggplant half with the veggie mixture and rice.

11. Drizzle with the dressing and sesame seeds, dividing equally. Refrigerate leftovers in an air-tight container for up to 4 days.

VARIATION TIP: If you don't have any turmeric-tahini dressing already prepared, you can simply thin out hummus with 2 to 3 tablespoons warm water and season to taste with freshly squeezed lemon juice and a spice blend, such as Tuscan seasoning or my DIY Taco Seasoning (page 198).

CHICKPEA, KALE, AND SWEET POTATO BOWLS

SERVES 4 | **PREP TIME:** 15 MINUTES | **COOK TIME:** 5 MINUTES

30-MINUTE MEAL | **ONE POT/PAN** | **LEFTOVER-FRIENDLY** | **NUT-FREE** | **VEGAN**

What could be simpler than a bowl of canned chickpeas and tofu, two common kitchen staples that don't even need to be cooked? If you like raw kale, you'll save yourself even more time with this recipe, although I find that a few extra minutes spent blanching and sautéing the kale are worth it.

4 cups chopped lacinato kale

4 teaspoons olive oil

½ teaspoon sea salt

2 medium sweet potatoes, sliced

¼ cup water

1½ cups canned chickpeas, drained and rinsed

1 pound firm tofu, chopped

¼ cup Turmeric-Tahini Dressing (page 195)

2 tablespoons chopped scallions, green parts only

PER SERVING (1 BOWL):
Calories: 375; Fat: 17g; Carbohydrates: 40g; Protein: 20g; Fiber: 11g; Sodium: 542mg; Iron: 52mg

1. Using your hands, massage the kale to break down its tough fibers. Season with the oil and salt. Divide among 4 bowls.

2. Put the sweet potatoes in a microwave-safe bowl with the water. Cover and microwave for 5 minutes, or until soft. Let cool.

3. Layer each bowl with the sweet potatoes, chickpeas, and tofu, dividing equally.

4. Drizzle with the dressing.

5. Garnish with the scallions and serve. Refrigerate leftovers in an airtight container for up to 3 days.

VARIATION TIP: Swap out the Turmeric-Tahini Dressing for an equal amount of Creamy Cilantro Dressing (page 194) and garnish with cilantro instead of scallions. You can also swap out the sweet potatoes for Sweet Potato Medallions (page 203) for a more flavor-infused sweet potato option.

MEDITERRANEAN BOWLS

SERVES 4 | PREP TIME: 10 MINUTES

30-MINUTE MEAL | ONE POT/PAN | NUT-FREE | VEGETARIAN

Leftovers or prepped-ahead batches of tabbouleh make these bowls a snap, but even if you don't have the salad already made, the tabbouleh is a quick and easy blend (you can even shortcut it further by swapping in frozen rice for the farro). Served over crisp romaine lettuce, this Mediterranean-inspired dish is quite refreshing.

4 cups chopped romaine lettuce

¼ cup freshly squeezed lemon juice

½ cup hummus, divided

2 cups Tabbouleh Salad with Farro (page 58), divided

8 medium pitted green olives, chopped

2 small cucumbers, chopped

4 ounces feta cheese crumbled

PER SERVING (1 BOWL):
Calories: 263; Fat: 17g; Carbohydrates: 22g; Protein: 9g; Fiber: 6g; Sodium: 607mg; Iron: 3mg

1. In a large bowl, combine the lettuce and lemon juice. Toss well. Divide among 4 bowls.
2. Layer with the hummus, tabbouleh, olives, cucumbers, and cheese, dividing equally. Serve immediately.

SUBSTITUTION TIP: Make this bowl vegan by swapping out the feta for a small sliced avocado.

BLACK BEAN FIESTA BOWLS

SERVES 6 | PREP TIME: 10 MINUTES **| COOK TIME:** 10 MINUTES

30-MINUTE MEAL | NUT-FREE | VEGETARIAN

You can almost create this festive dish straight from the cupboard. Black beans, a good source of protein and fiber, are a great staple to have stocked. DIY taco seasoning is a cinch to make with just four common spices (you'll have enough to store for future uses). And sautéing onion and bell peppers couldn't be easier.

3 tablespoons olive oil

2 cups chopped yellow onion

½ teaspoon sea salt

3 cups frozen tricolor bell pepper strips, thawed

3 cups canned low-sodium black beans, drained and rinsed

2 tablespoons DIY Taco Seasoning (page 198)

2 cups frozen sweet corn

6 cups chopped romaine lettuce

1½ tablespoons freshly squeezed lemon juice

6 tablespoons Creamy Cilantro Dressing (page 194)

1. In a large skillet, heat the oil over medium heat for 30 seconds.

2. Add the onion, salt, and bell pepper. Sauté for 7 minutes, or until the veggies are soft and the onion is translucent.

3. Meanwhile, in a small bowl, combine the beans and taco seasoning. Mix well.

4. Move the onions and bell peppers to the sides of the skillet. Add the beans and corn directly over the heat, cooking until warmed through. Stir together the onion, bell pepper, beans, and corn. Remove from the heat.

5. Divide the lettuce evenly among 6 bowls.

6. Drizzle with the lemon juice.

7. Top each bowl with an equal amount of the bean mixture and 1 tablespoon of cilantro dressing.

PER SERVING (1 BOWL): Calories: 319; Fat: 11g; Carbohydrates: 49g; Protein: 12g; Fiber: 15g; Sodium: 454mg; Iron: 4mg

VARIATION TIP: Instead of the Creamy Cilantro Dressing, you can use an equal amount of Avocado-Dill Dressing (page 196). Add a tablespoon of Crispy Chickpeas (page 201) or toasted walnuts for more crunch.

QUINOA HARVEST BOWLS

SERVES 4 | **PREP TIME:** 20 MINUTES | **COOK TIME:** 45 MINUTES

LEFTOVER-FRIENDLY | **GLUTEN-FREE** | **VEGETARIAN**

These harvest quinoa bowls are assembled with colorful root veggies, peppery arugula, and a tangy Dijon vinaigrette.

1 medium beet, scrubbed

Nonstick cooking spray, for coating

½ cup quinoa

1 cup chopped carrots

1½ cups water

⅜ teaspoon sea salt, divided

1 tablespoon balsamic vinegar

1 teaspoon Dijon mustard

½ teaspoon honey

2 tablespoons olive oil

1 cup low-sodium canned chickpeas, drained and rinsed

1 cup arugula

3 tablespoons dried cranberries

¼ cup chopped walnuts

PER SERVING (¼ RECIPE):
Calories: 308; Fat: 15g; Carbohydrates: 39g; Protein: 8g; Fiber: 7g; Sodium: 245mg; Iron: 2mg

1. Preheat the oven to 400°F.
2. Coat the beet with cooking spray and wrap tightly in aluminum foil. Place on a baking sheet.
3. Transfer the baking sheet to the oven, and bake for 45 minutes, or until the beet is soft. Remove from the oven. Let cool for 10 minutes.
4. Meanwhile, in a medium saucepan, combine the quinoa, carrots, water, and ⅛ teaspoon of salt. Bring to a boil over medium-high heat.
5. Reduce the heat to medium-low. Cover the saucepan and simmer for 15 minutes, or until the water has been absorbed. Remove from the heat. Stir in ⅛ teaspoon of salt.
6. Once the beet is cool enough to handle, pull away the skin, using the foil to catch it (it should easily slide away). Finely dice the beet.
7. To make the dressing, in a small bowl, whisk together the vinegar, mustard, honey, oil, and remaining ⅛ teaspoon of salt.
8. In a medium bowl, combine the quinoa-carrot mixture, roasted beet, chickpeas, arugula, cranberries, and walnuts.
9. Mix in the dressing and serve. Refrigerate leftovers in an airtight container for up to 3 days.

TECHNICAL TIP: Adding salt after cooking helps flavor the quinoa.

GINGER-SOY NOODLE BOWLS

SERVES 4 | PREP TIME: 10 MINUTES **| COOK TIME:** 15 MINUTES

30-MINUTE MEAL | LEFTOVER-FRIENDLY | VEGETARIAN

These noodle bowls are made with ramen noodles, which are ready in just 3 minutes. Save a little pasta water to help the sauce better adhere to the noodles.

¼ teaspoon salt

6¼ cups water, divided

4 cups chopped curly kale

2 (3-ounce) packages instant ramen noodles, spice packets discarded

¾ cup Sesame Dressing (page 193)

2 tablespoons chopped scallions, green parts only

2 teaspoons olive oil, divided

2 or 3 garlic cloves, minced

2 cups small broccoli florets

1 cup shredded carrots

1 medium, ripe avocado, pitted, peeled, and sliced

8 ounces firm tofu, cut into ½-inch cubes

2 tablespoons sliced almonds

PER SERVING (1 MACRO BOWL): Calories: 508; Fat: 34g; Carbohydrates: 39g; Protein: 16g; Fiber: 8g; Sodium: 836mg; Iron: 4mg

1. In a large soup pot, salt 6 cups of water. Bring to a boil over high heat.

2. Add the kale and cook until it begins to soften, 1 to 2 minutes. Using a slotted spoon, remove promptly (saving the water to cook the noodles) and rinse with cold water.

3. Add the noodles to the pot and cook them over high heat for 3 minutes, or until tender. Remove from the heat. Transfer to a bowl with 1 tablespoon of the pasta cooking water.

4. Add the dressing and scallions. Stir to mix.

5. In a small skillet, heat 1 teaspoon of oil over medium heat for 30 seconds.

6. Add the garlic and stir for 1 minute, or until crisp and golden. Remove from the heat.

7. In a microwave-safe dish, combine the broccoli with the remaining ¼ cup of water. Cover and microwave for 4 minutes, or until tender. Drain any excess water.

8. Divide the seasoned noodles, broccoli, kale, carrots, avocado, and tofu among 4 bowls.

9. Drizzle the remaining 1 teaspoon of oil over the broccoli.

10. Garnish the kale with the crisp garlic.

11. Sprinkle on the almonds. Serve.

CURRIED LENTIL STEW

SERVES 4 | PREP TIME: 10 MINUTES | **COOK TIME:** 55 MINUTES TO 1 HOUR
LEFTOVER-FRIENDLY | NUT-FREE | VEGAN

A complete meal, this stew has your veggies, starch, plenty of protein, and fiber, too! With a curry flavor that's savory but not too hot, here is a comforting meal the whole family can enjoy.

¾ cup dried brown lentils, rinsed

3¼ cups water, divided

2 teaspoons olive oil

2 cups 5-Ingredient Mirepoix (page 199)

1½ teaspoons curry powder

1 medium, vine-ripened tomato, sliced

2 tablespoons tomato paste

2 tablespoons all-purpose flour

1¼ cups low-sodium vegetable broth

1 teaspoon low-sodium soy sauce

1½ cups diced peeled butternut squash

4 cups chopped chard

PER SERVING (1½ CUPS):
Calories: 245; Fat: 3g; Carbohydrates: 45g; Protein: 13g; Fiber: 8g; Sodium: 326mg; Iron: 4mg

1. In a medium saucepan, combine the lentils and 2¼ cups of water. Bring to a boil over medium heat.

2. Reduce the heat to low. Cover the saucepan and simmer for 12 to 14 minutes, or until the lentils are tender. Remove from the heat. Drain.

3. Once the lentils have cooked for about 5 minutes, in a medium soup pot, heat the oil over medium-high heat for 30 seconds.

4. Add the mirepoix. Reduce the heat to medium. Stir and cook for 7 minutes, or until the veggies are tender.

5. Stir in the curry powder and cook for 1 to 2 minutes, or until fragrant.

6. Add the tomato, tomato paste, flour, broth, soy sauce, remaining 1 cup of water, the squash, and lentils. Stir well.

7. Reduce the heat to medium-low. Cover the pot and cook for 25 minutes, or until the squash is tender.

8. Add the chard, cover the pot again, and cook the chard for 10 minutes, or until wilted. Remove from the heat. Serve. Refrigerate leftovers in an airtight container for up to a week. Like soups, the flavors of this curry come together over time and taste even better the second time around.

VEGGIE BURGER PARMESAN

SERVES 4 | **PREP TIME:** 10 MINUTES, PLUS 30 MINUTES TO CHILL | **COOK TIME:** 25 MINUTES

LEFTOVER-FRIENDLY | NUT-FREE | VEGETARIAN

A veggie-inspired version of chicken parmesan requires no egg batter or coating (which also means less time and fewer dishes). You'll enjoy these veggies smothered in a zesty marinara with zucchini and spinach and topped with parmesan for a comforting vegetarian meal. Clean your plate by soaking up any remaining marinara with the bread.

1 cup rolled oats

1½ cups canned chickpeas, drained and rinsed

½ cup frozen peas

½ cup shredded carrots

1 medium egg

2 teaspoons low-sodium, vegan Worcestershire sauce or low-sodium soy sauce

2 teaspoons olive oil, plus 1 tablespoon

4 cups thinly sliced zucchini or yellow squash

1 tablespoon Tuscan seasoning

1 cup marinara sauce

1 cup baby spinach

4 tablespoons grated parmesan cheese

1 sourdough toast slice, cut into 4 equal wedges

1. Prepare the veggie burgers: in a food processor, combine the oats, chickpeas, peas, and carrots. Process until the mixture is well ground but some small chunks of veggies are still visible. Transfer to a medium bowl.

2. Mix in the egg and Worcestershire sauce. Form into 3-inch patties. Place in a single layer on a large plate. Cover and refrigerate for 30 minutes.

3. In a large skillet, heat 2 teaspoons of oil over medium-high heat for 30 seconds.

4. When it shimmers, carefully add the zucchini and Tuscan seasoning. Toss to coat, then spread out evenly in the skillet.

5. Reduce the heat to medium. Cook for 7 minutes, or until the bottoms of the zucchini slices are lightly browned.

6. Add the marinara; toss and cook for another 7 minutes, or until the zucchini is tender.

7. Mix in the spinach until wilted. Remove from the heat. Transfer the entire mixture to a bowl. Use a heatproof silicone spatula to scrape the skillet as clean as possible.

8. Using the same skillet, heat the remaining 1 tablespoon of oil over medium heat for 1 minute, or until shimmering.

9. Add the patties and cook for 4 to 6 minutes per side, or until browned. Remove from the heat.

10. Serve one-fourth of the marinara-zucchini mixture over each patty with 1 tablespoon of cheese and a wedge of sourdough toast for dipping.

VARIATION TIP: Tuscan seasoning can have just enough red pepper flakes to create some heat. To keep it on the mild side, use an equal amount of Italian seasoning instead.

PER SERVING (¼ OF THE RECIPE): Calories: 393; Fat: 14g; Carbohydrates: 55g; Protein: 16g; Fiber: 10g; Sodium: 665mg; Iron: 5mg

VEGGIE MEATLOAF

SERVES 6 | **PREP TIME:** 15 MINUTES, PLUS 30 MINUTES TO CHILL | **COOK TIME:** 1 HOUR

LEFTOVER-FRIENDLY | **NUT-FREE** | **VEGETARIAN**

When you want some good comfort food, this meatloaf is guaranteed to hit the spot—and it's vegetarian to boot. With a flavorful mirepoix as a veggie-centric filler, you've got all you need to hold the loaf together. Nutrient-rich lentils provide most of the fiber and protein in this meatless dish.

1 cup dried brown lentils, rinsed

3¼ cups water, divided

2 teaspoons olive oil, plus 1 tablespoon

2 cups 5-Ingredient Mirepoix (page 199)

¾ cup panko bread crumbs

1 tablespoon garlic powder or DIY Taco Seasoning (page 198)

1 medium egg

½ cup Date-Sweetened Barbecue Sauce (page 191), divided

3 medium russet potatoes, scrubbed and rinsed

½ cup plain low-fat Greek yogurt

¼ teaspoon sea salt

2 cups fresh or frozen green beans, trimmed

PER SERVING (⅙ OF THE RECIPE): Calories: 333; Fat: 6g; Carbohydrates: 60g; Protein: 15g; Fiber: 11g; Sodium: 204mg; Iron: 5mg

1. Preheat the oven to 350°F. Line a 5-by-9-inch loaf pan with parchment paper.

2. In a medium saucepan, combine the lentils and 3 cups of water. Bring to a boil over medium heat.

3. Reduce the heat to low. Cover the saucepan and simmer for 12 to 14 minutes, or until the lentils are tender. Remove from the heat. Drain.

4. Meanwhile, in a medium skillet, heat 2 teaspoons of oil over medium heat for 30 seconds.

5. Add the mirepoix and sauté for 7 minutes, or until the veggies are soft. Remove from the heat. Transfer to a medium bowl.

6. Mix in the lentils, bread crumbs, garlic powder, egg, and ¼ cup of barbecue sauce. Mold the mixture into the prepared loaf pan. Cover and refrigerate for 30 minutes.

7. Coat with the remaining ¼ cup of barbecue sauce.

8. Transfer the loaf pan to the oven and bake for 45 minutes, or until the loaf is firm and a toothpick inserted into the center comes out clean. Remove from the oven. Let cool for 5 minutes.

9. Meanwhile, boil the potatoes. Put the potatoes in a medium soup pot with enough water to cover them fully. Bring to a boil over medium-high heat. Cook for 30 minutes, or until tender. Remove from the heat. Drain and return the potatoes to the pot.

10. Add the remaining 1 tablespoon of oil, the yogurt, and salt. Mash.

11. In a microwave-safe bowl, combine the green beans and remaining ¼ cup of water. Cover and microwave for 4 minutes, or until tender. Drain any excess water.

12. Serve the meatloaf over the potatoes with green beans on the side. Refrigerate leftover meatloaf in an airtight container for 3 to 4 days.

TECHNICAL TIP: Chilling the loaf mixture for 30 minutes prior to cooking helps it stay firm and prevents crumbling, creating a better overall texture.

VEGETARIAN SHEPHERD'S PIE

SERVES 4 | **PREP TIME:** 10 MINUTES | **COOK TIME:** 1 HOUR

LEFTOVER-FRIENDLY | **NUT-FREE** | **VEGETARIAN**

Who said shepherd's pie can't be vegetarian? This version of the classic is made with a savory seasoned lentil blend and creamy mashed potatoes. It's simpler than you may think, too. Instant mashed potatoes will save you cooking time, and lentils are a relatively quick-cooking legume.

Nonstick cooking spray, for coating

1 cup dried brown lentils, rinsed

5 cups water, divided

2 teaspoons olive oil

1 recipe 5-Ingredient Mirepoix (page 199)

2 garlic cloves, minced

2 tablespoons all-purpose flour

1 cup low-fat (1 percent) milk, divided

¼ cup tomato paste

1¼ teaspoons curry powder, divided (or Italian seasoning for a milder version)

1½ tablespoons low-sodium soy sauce

2 cups baby spinach

1 cup instant mashed potatoes

1. Preheat the oven to 350°F. Lightly grease a 9-by-9-inch baking dish with cooking spray.

2. In a medium saucepan, combine the lentils and 3 cups of water. Bring to a boil over medium heat.

3. Reduce the heat to low. Cover the saucepan and simmer for 12 to 14 minutes, or until the lentils are tender. Remove from the heat. Drain.

4. In a large skillet, heat the olive oil over medium heat for 30 seconds.

5. Add the mirepoix and garlic. Sauté, stirring occasionally, for 7 minutes, or until the veggies are soft.

6. Add the lentils, flour, ⅔ cup of milk, the tomato paste, 1 teaspoon of curry powder, and the soy sauce. Mix until well incorporated.

7. Fold in the spinach and cook until it starts to wilt. Remove from the heat. Transfer to the prepared baking dish.

8. Pour the remaining 2 cups of water into the same skillet. Bring to a boil over medium-high heat.

9. Add the instant potatoes. Reduce the heat to medium. Stir for about 1 minute, or until thickened. Remove from the heat.

10. Mix in the remaining ⅓ cup of milk and ¼ teaspoon of curry powder.

11. Carefully spread the mashed potatoes over the lentil mixture in the baking dish. Lightly coat the top with cooking spray.

12. Transfer the baking dish to the oven and bake for 25 to 30 minutes, or until lightly browned and slightly crisp on the surface. You may need to broil for 3 minutes if you do not achieve a golden color after baking. Remove from the oven. Refrigerate leftovers in an airtight container for up to 4 days.

SUBSTITUTION TIP: To make this vegan, swap out the milk for ½ cup low-sodium vegetable broth and ½ cup water (mixed together to reduce sodium). Or use a blend of ¾ cup water and ¼ cup Date-Sweetened Teriyaki Sauce (page 190), which pairs excellently with the curry flavor.

PER SERVING (¼ OF THE RECIPE—ABOUT 1 CUP): Calories: 323; Fat: 4g; Carbohydrates: 57g; Protein: 17g; Fiber: 11g; Sodium: 586mg; Iron: 5mg

ROASTED VEGGIE MAC-N-CHEESE AU GRATIN

SERVES 4 | **PREP TIME:** 10 MINUTES | **COOK TIME:** 30 MINUTES

LEFTOVER-FRIENDLY | **NUT-FREE** | **VEGETARIAN**

It may be a classic, kid-friendly comfort meal, but this mac-n-cheese au gratin has plenty of protein, fiber, and veggies for a nourishing dish both adults and kids will enjoy. Reheat leftovers in the oven at 350°F for about 15 minutes to retain the crispness of the panko crust.

Nonstick cooking spray, for coating

8 ounces dried macaroni noodles (such as thick elbow noodles)

¼ cup panko bread crumbs

2 cups shredded cheddar cheese, divided

1 tablespoon grated parmesan cheese

1 teaspoon Italian seasoning

2 teaspoons olive oil

2 tablespoons all-purpose flour

¼ teaspoon garlic powder

⅛ teaspoon sea salt

¾ cup low-fat (1 percent) milk

2 cups frozen peas and carrots, thawed, divided

1. Preheat the oven to 350°F. Lightly grease a 9-by-13-inch baking dish with cooking spray.

2. Cook the noodles according to the package instructions. Reserve 2 tablespoons of pasta water before draining.

3. Pour the cooked noodles and reserved pasta water into the prepared baking dish.

4. Meanwhile, in a small bowl, combine the bread crumbs, ¼ cup of cheddar cheese, the parmesan cheese, and Italian seasoning.

5. In a medium saucepan over medium heat, whisk together the olive oil, flour, garlic powder, salt, and milk until the mixture starts to thicken.

6. Stir in the remaining 1¾ cups of cheddar cheese until well incorporated. Remove from the heat. Pour the cheese sauce over the noodles, then mix in 1 cup of the peas and carrots.

7. Evenly sprinkle the bread crumb mixture on top of the macaroni in the baking dish. Coat with cooking spray.

8. Transfer the baking dish to the oven and bake for 15 to 20 minutes, or until the mac-n-cheese has lightly browned. Remove from the oven.

9. Serve the mac-n-cheese with the remaining 1 cup of peas and carrots on the side.

TECHNICAL TIP: Using a little pasta water helps the cheese sauce stick to the pasta better.

PER SERVING (¼ OF THE RECIPE—ABOUT 1 CUP): Calories: 443; Fat: 22g; Carbohydrates: 41g; Protein: 22g; Fiber: 4g; Sodium: 645mg; Iron: 2mg

SPAGHETTI AND VEGETARIAN "MEAT"BALLS

SERVES 4 | **PREP TIME:** 5 MINUTES, PLUS 30 MINUTES TO CHILL | **COOK TIME:** 30 MINUTES

LEFTOVER-FRIENDLY | **NUT-FREE** | **VEGETARIAN**

Hearty and fiber-rich, these plant-based meatballs are flavorful and satisfying. Serve over pasta with marinara. You won't miss the beef.

Nonstick cooking spray, for coating the baking sheet

2 teaspoons olive oil

⅓ cup 5-Ingredient Mirepoix (page 199) or chopped yellow onions

2 garlic cloves, minced

1½ cups low-sodium canned black beans, drained and rinsed

1 tablespoon DIY Taco Seasoning (page 198)

1 cup panko bread crumbs

1 medium egg

¼ cup tomato paste

¼ cup chopped scallions, green parts only

8 ounces spaghetti

1 cup marinara sauce

2 cups frozen green beans

¼ cup water

PER SERVING (¼ OF THE RECIPE): Calories: 391; Fat: 7g; Carbohydrates: 71g; Protein: 16g; Fiber: 15g; Sodium: 517mg; Iron: 5mg

1. Preheat the oven to 350°F. Lightly grease a rimmed baking sheet or a 9-by-9-inch baking dish with cooking spray.

2. In a medium skillet, heat the olive oil over medium heat for 30 seconds.

3. Add the mirepoix and garlic. Sauté, stirring occasionally, for 7 minutes, or until the veggies are soft. Remove from the heat.

4. To make the batter, in a medium mixing bowl, combine the beans, taco seasoning, bread crumbs, egg, tomato paste, scallions, and mirepoix mixture. Using a fork, mash until well combined. Cover and chill in the refrigerator for 30 minutes.

5. Scoop the batter into 1½-inch balls and place them on the prepared baking sheet.

6. Transfer the baking sheet to the oven and bake for 20 minutes, or until the meatballs are firm. Remove from the oven.

7. Meanwhile, cook the spaghetti according to the package instructions.

8. In a microwave-safe bowl, combine the green beans and water. Cover and microwave for 4 minutes, or until tender. Drain any excess water.

9. Serve 3 meatballs over ½ cup of spaghetti and ¼ cup of marinara, with ½ cup of green beans on the side, per serving.

VARIATION TIP: If you've got any Date-Sweetened Teriyaki Sauce (page 190) on hand, use it in place of the tomato paste for an extra kick of flavor. The pungency of the ginger and garlic and the saltiness of the soy sauce complement the zesty tomato sauce nicely for an umami appeal. (Note: You may need to add a tablespoon or two more panko to maintain the right meatball consistency, since the teriyaki sauce is thinner.)

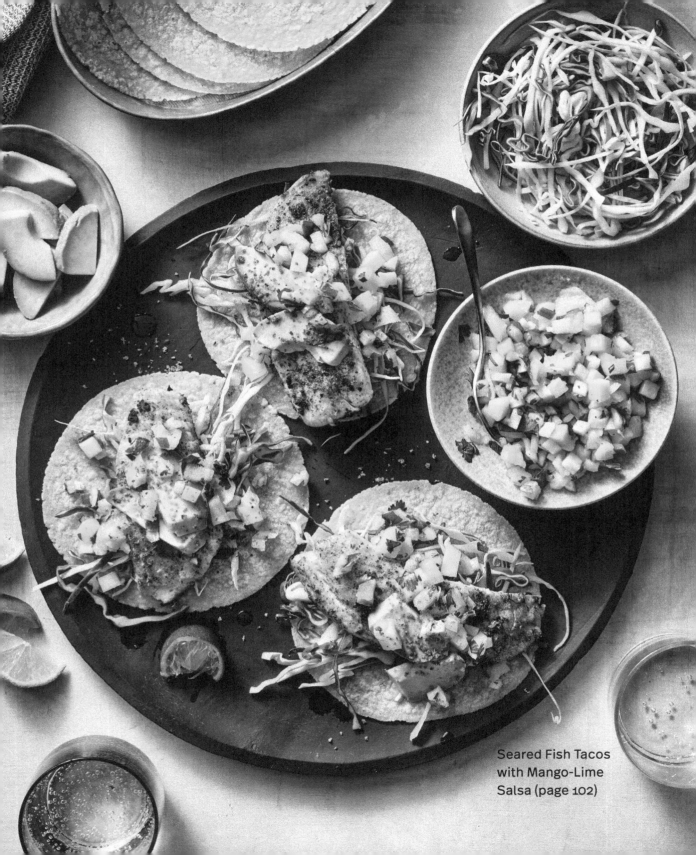

Seared Fish Tacos with Mango-Lime Salsa (page 102)

CHAPTER 6

FISH AND SEAFOOD

Tuna Toasts with
Lemon-Caper Aïoli **96**

Sesame Avocado Salad
with Tuna **97**

Shrimp and Arugula
Salad **98**

One-Pot Taco Shrimp **99**

Shrimp and Grits over
Collard Greens **100**

Seared Fish Tacos with
Mango-Lime Salsa **102**

Pan-Seared Tilapia over
Lemon-Parmesan Pasta **104**

Mexican-Inspired Tilapia
with Bell Peppers and
Kale **106**

Foil-Wrapped Tuscan
Haddock **107**

Haddock with Creamy
Yogurt Mayonnaise **108**

Tahini Roasted Salmon with
Warm Kale Salad **110**

Baked Salmon with Creamy
Cilantro Dressing **112**

Teriyaki Salmon Bowls **113**

Avocado-Dill Poached
Salmon **114**

Sesame Salmon Protein
Bowls **116**

TUNA TOASTS WITH LEMON-CAPER AÏOLI

SERVES 4 | PREP TIME: 10 MINUTES

30-MINUTE MEAL | LEFTOVER-FRIENDLY | NUT-FREE

Lemon-caper aïoli is a great alternative to traditional mayonnaise in a tuna salad. With Dijon, lemon, capers, and garlic, it's creamy, delicious, and delightfully pungent, giving this tuna salad a gourmet feel.

4 whole-grain bread slices

4 (4-ounce) cans water-packed tuna, drained

½ cup Lemon-Caper Aïoli (page 197)

4 cups arugula

4 teaspoons olive oil

⅛ teaspoon sea salt

Juice of ½ lemon

2 tablespoons grated parmesan cheese

1. Toast the bread in a toaster or toaster oven.
2. Meanwhile, flake the tuna into a bowl with the aïoli. Mix well, then divide evenly among the toasts.
3. In a medium bowl, toss together the arugula, oil, salt, and lemon juice.
4. Garnish with the cheese.
5. Serve the tuna toasts with the salad on the side. Refrigerate leftover tuna salad in an airtight container for 3 to 4 days.

PER SERVING (1 OPEN-FACE SANDWICH WITH SIDE SALAD): Calories: 265; Fat: 11g; Carbohydrates: 16g; Protein: 27g; Fiber: 3g; Sodium: 735mg; Iron: 3mg

VARIATION TIP: Replace the toast with a whole-wheat tortilla and serve as a wrap.

SESAME AVOCADO SALAD WITH TUNA

SERVES 4 | PREP TIME: 5 MINUTES

30-MINUTE MEAL

Sesame seeds add a light, toasty crunch to the creaminess of avocado, a textural pairing that's oh-so-satisfying in this salad. With crisp romaine lettuce and sesame dressing, this simple salad packs in plenty of flavor. Because of their crunch, rice cakes are a great swap for traditional fried wonton noodles.

2 (4-ounce) cans water-packed tuna, drained

Juice of 1 medium lemon

¼ teaspoon garlic powder

1 medium, ripe avocado, pitted, peeled, and chopped

1 cup shredded carrots

1 cup sliced mushrooms

4 cups chopped romaine lettuce

½ cup Sesame Dressing (page 193)

2 tablespoons toasted sesame seeds

4 rice cakes

PER SERVING (¼ OF THE RECIPE): Calories: 300; Fat: 16g; Carbohydrates: 22g; Protein: 19g; Fiber: 6g; Sodium: 199mg; Iron: 3mg

1. Flake the tuna into a medium bowl.
2. Add the lemon juice and garlic powder. Mix well.
3. Reserve a few pieces of avocado, carrots, and mushrooms for garnish. In a large salad bowl, toss together the remaining pieces with the lettuce.
4. Add the dressing and toss again to coat.
5. Garnish with the reserved avocado, carrots, and mushrooms.
6. Top with the sesame seeds.
7. Serve each portion with 2 ounces of tuna on top and a rice cake either on the side or crumbled on top for garnish.

VARIATION TIP: Add ¼ cup sliced Ginger Pickled Radish (page 200) for more color and to make this salad even zestier.

SHRIMP AND ARUGULA SALAD

SERVES 4 | PREP TIME: 10 MINUTES | **COOK TIME:** 10 MINUTES

30-MINUTE MEAL | LEFTOVER-FRIENDLY | GLUTEN-FREE | NUT-FREE

This salad is a perfectly light meal, easily assembled with three of my favorite veggie staples—edamame, carrots, and avocado—and the deliciously tangy lemon-caper aïoli.

1 pound medium raw frozen shrimp, peeled, deveined, tails removed

2 teaspoons olive oil

4 cups arugula

1 cup shelled edamame

1 cup shredded carrots

½ cup Lemon-Caper Aïoli (page 197)

1 medium, ripe avocado, pitted, peeled, and diced

PER SERVING (¼ OF THE RECIPE): Calories: 232; Fat: 11g; Carbohydrates: 14g; Protein: 22g; Fiber: 6g; Sodium: 549mg; Iron: 2mg

1. Thaw the shrimp: in a large bowl, submerge the shrimp in cold water while gently running cool water over the top for 5 to 10 minutes, or until the shrimp is pliable. Drain.

2. In a nonstick skillet, heat the oil over medium-high heat for 30 seconds.

3. Add the shrimp and sauté for 2 to 3 minutes per side, or until the shrimp is pink and no longer translucent. Remove from the heat.

4. In a large bowl, toss together the arugula, edamame, and carrots.

5. Fold in the shrimp and toss with the aïoli until well coated.

6. Divide the salad evenly among 4 bowls.

7. Garnish each bowl with the avocado.

VARIATION TIP: If you prefer to grill the shrimp, preheat your grill to medium, place the shrimp on skewers, and lightly coat them with cooking spray. Grill for 2 to 3 minutes per side, or until blackened.

ONE-POT TACO SHRIMP

SERVES 4 | PREP TIME: 15 MINUTES **| COOK TIME:** 15 TO 20 MINUTES
NUT-FREE

Using the same pot for all your cooking transfers the seasoning to every component of the dish. It will save you cleanup time, too!

1 pound medium raw frozen shrimp, peeled, deveined, tails removed

1 tablespoon olive oil

1 tablespoon DIY Taco Seasoning (page 198)

2 cups frozen tricolor bell pepper strips

4 cups water

¼ teaspoon sea salt

1⅓ cups dried couscous

4 cups baby spinach

PER SERVING (¼ OF THE RECIPE): Calories: 347; Fat: 5g; Carbohydrates: 52g; Protein: 22g; Fiber: 7g; Sodium: 620mg; Iron: 3mg

1. Thaw the shrimp: in a large bowl, submerge the shrimp in cold water while gently running cool water over the top for about 5 to 10 minutes, or until the shrimp is pliable. Drain.

2. In a medium soup pot, heat the oil over medium-high heat for 30 seconds.

3. Reduce the heat to medium. Add the taco seasoning and toast for 30 seconds, or until fragrant.

4. Add the shrimp and bell pepper. Sauté for 2 to 3 minutes per side, or until the shrimp is pink and no longer translucent and the bell pepper has warmed through. Remove to a plate.

5. In the same pot, bring the water and salt to a boil over high heat.

6. Reduce the heat to medium. Add the couscous. Cover the pot and simmer for 6 minutes, or until the couscous is tender. Remove from the heat. Drain any excess water.

7. Plate the couscous over the spinach.

8. Top with the shrimp and bell peppers. Serve immediately.

VARIATION TIP: For a different texture, swap out the couscous for instant grits or angel hair pasta; they all take around the same time to cook.

SHRIMP AND GRITS OVER COLLARD GREENS

SERVES 4 | **PREP TIME:** 15 MINUTES | **COOK TIME:** 25 TO 30 MINUTES

GLUTEN-FREE | **NUT-FREE**

The garlic-infused oil in these shrimp and grits permeates through-out the dish. It's an easy Southern-style meal that you can make in just minutes and that will satisfy your whole family.

1 pound medium raw frozen shrimp, peeled, deveined, tails removed

1½ tablespoons olive oil

4 teaspoons minced garlic

8 cups stemmed and chopped collard greens, rinsed and wrung dry

4 cups water

¼ teaspoon sea salt

1 cup instant yellow grits

PER SERVING (¼ OF THE RECIPE): Calories: 207; Fat: 6g; Carbohydrates: 15g; Protein: 19g; Fiber: 5g; Sodium: 536mg; Iron: 5mg

1. Thaw the shrimp: in a large bowl, submerge the shrimp in cold water while gently running cool water over the top for about 5 to 10 minutes, or until the shrimp is pliable. Drain.

2. In a large, high-sided pan or soup pot, heat the oil over medium-high heat for 1 minute, or until shimmering.

3. Add the garlic and cook for 30 seconds, or until fragrant. Remove from the pan.

4. Add the collard greens and cook, stirring occasionally, for 8 to 10 minutes, or until tender, bright, and wilted. Transfer the greens to a large serving platter and mix in half of the cooked garlic.

5. Add the shrimp and remaining cooked garlic to the pan. Sauté for 2 to 3 minutes per side, or until the shrimp is pink and no longer trans-lucent. Remove from the pan and lay on top of the greens.

6. Add the water to the pan. Increase the heat to high. Add the salt and bring to a boil.

7. Reduce the heat to low. Slowly stir in the grits. Cook, stirring occasionally to prevent large lumps, for 5 to 6 minutes, or until the water has been absorbed. Remove from the heat.
8. Divide the grits evenly among 4 plates. Top with the greens and shrimp. Serve immediately.

TECHNICAL TIP: To prevent browning residue on the bottom of the pan as you cook, add low-sodium chicken broth, 1 tablespoon at a time. Keep a watchful eye on the grits, scraping the bottom of the pan as you cook and stirring occasionally with a spatula.

SEARED FISH TACOS WITH MANGO-LIME SALSA

SERVES 4 | **PREP TIME:** 15 MINUTES | **COOK TIME:** 10 MINUTES

30-MINUTE MEAL | **LEFTOVER-FRIENDLY** | **GLUTEN-FREE** | **NUT-FREE**

Fish tacos make for a simple, family-friendly meal. This version uses a fresh mango salsa with lime for a tangy, sweet appeal. For best results, prepare the salsa at least three hours ahead of time and refrigerate in an airtight container to let the flavors meld.

For the salsa

1 cup diced mango

¼ cup chopped fennel bulb

2 tablespoons chopped red onion

Juice of 1 lime

⅛ teaspoon sea salt

2 tablespoons chopped fresh cilantro

For the tacos

1 tablespoon olive oil

2 (6-ounce) tilapia fillets, patted dry

¼ teaspoon sea salt

½ teaspoon ground cumin

Grated zest of 1 lime

8 (6-inch) corn tortillas

1 cup shredded cabbage

1 medium, ripe avocado, pitted, peeled, and sliced

¼ teaspoon Tajín chili-lime seasoning

To make the salsa

1. In a medium bowl, toss together the mango, fennel, onion, lime juice, salt, and cilantro until well combined.

To make the tacos

2. In a large sealable bag, combine the oil, tilapia, salt, cumin, and lime zest. Shake well to coat.

3. Heat a medium skillet over medium heat for 1 minute, or until warmed.

4. Add the coated tilapia. Cook for 3 to 4 minutes per side, or until the fish flakes easily. Remove from the heat. Transfer the tilapia to a plate and flake it into chunks.

5. Place 4 sets of 2 stacked tortillas on a cutting board.

6. Layer each stack with ¼ cup of cabbage and a few slices of avocado.

7. Sprinkle the Tajín seasoning on top.

8. Divide the tilapia and salsa evenly among the tacos. Fold and enjoy! Refrigerate leftovers in an airtight container for 3 days.

TECHNICAL TIP: To cut a mango, use a sharp chef's knife and a solid cutting board to avoid slippage. Positioning the mango upright, cut along the widest, flattest sides first to create 2 thick slices. Then cut the remaining 2 sides. Cut each section into long lengthwise slits, then turn it 90 degrees to make similar size slits to form a criss-cross pattern. Scoop out mango cubes with a spoon.

PER SERVING (1 TACO): Calories: 355; Fat: 13g; Carbohydrates: 38g; Protein: 27g; Fiber: 8g; Sodium: 287mg; Iron: 2mg

PAN-SEARED TILAPIA OVER LEMON-PARMESAN PASTA

SERVES 4 | **PREP TIME:** 5 MINUTES | **COOK TIME:** 15 MINUTES

30-MINUTE MEAL | **NUT-FREE**

Pan-searing creates a tasty crust on the fish, and because it's cooked at a higher heat, it takes just minutes to prepare. This dish has the best of both creamy and crisp with a delicate sauce that coats the pasta.

2 tablespoons olive oil, divided

3 garlic cloves, minced

4 cups chopped kale or collard greens

2 (6-ounce) tilapia fillets, halved

¼ teaspoon lemon pepper seasoning

Juice of 1 lemon

1 tablespoon all-purpose flour

½ cup low-fat (1 percent) milk

2 to 4 tablespoons water

8 ounces angel hair pasta

¼ teaspoon sea salt

¼ cup grated parmesan cheese

PER SERVING (¼ OF THE RECIPE): Calories: 421; Fat: 11g; Carbohydrates: 50g; Protein: 32g; Fiber: 3g; Sodium: 255mg; Iron: 3mg

1. Fill a large pot halfway with water. Bring to a boil over high heat.

2. Meanwhile, in a medium nonstick skillet, heat 1 tablespoon of oil over medium-high heat for 30 seconds.

3. Add the garlic to the skillet and cook for 30 seconds, or until fragrant.

4. Stir the kale into the skillet. Reduce the heat to medium. Cook for 2 minutes, or until the greens begin to wilt.

5. Push the veggies to the sides of the skillet. Add the tilapia and sear for 3 minutes per side.

6. Reduce the heat to low. Transfer the kale and tilapia to a plate. Season the tilapia with the lemon pepper.

7. Deglaze the skillet with the lemon juice.

8. Increase the heat to medium-low. Add the remaining 1 tablespoon of oil, the flour, and milk, stirring constantly as the mixture thickens into a sauce.

9. Add the water, 1 tablespoon at a time, to thin the sauce to your desired consistency if necessary.

10. Add the pasta to the boiling water and cook for 6 minutes, or until tender. Remove from the heat. Reserving 1 tablespoon of pasta cooking water, drain.

11. Add the reserved pasta water to the sauce and mix.

12. Add the pasta and toss to thoroughly coat. Remove from the heat.

13. Serve the tilapia and greens over the creamy pasta. Season with the salt.

14. Garnish with the cheese.

TECHNICAL TIP: You want the sauce to be thick enough to adhere well to the pasta. If the sauce is too watery at any point, add 1 to 2 teaspoons flour to the mix and continue to stir. If the sauce is too thick, you can always stir in a little water to thin it out.

MEXICAN-INSPIRED TILAPIA WITH BELL PEPPERS AND KALE

SERVES 6 | **PREP TIME:** 5 MINUTES | **COOK TIME:** 20 MINUTES

30-MINUTE MEAL | **GLUTEN-FREE** | **NUT-FREE**

Give your dinner a little heat and zest with this taco-style crusted tilapia. Pan-seared and served over grits with veggies, it's a simple, tasty meal that's got plenty of zip.

1½ cups instant
   yellow grits

3 tablespoons olive oil

3 tablespoons DIY
   Taco Seasoning
   (page 198), divided

6 (4-ounce) tilapia fillets

6 cups chopped kale

3 cups frozen tricolor bell
   pepper strips

PER SERVING (⅙ OF THE RECIPE): Calories: 347; Fat: 11g; Carbohydrates: 31g; Protein: 33g; Fiber: 6g; Sodium: 694mg; Iron: 13mg

1. Prepare the grits according to the package instructions. Cover the cooked grits to keep them warm.

2. In a medium nonstick skillet, heat the oil over medium-high heat for 30 seconds.

3. Stir in 1½ tablespoons of taco seasoning and cook for 1 minute, or until fragrant.

4. Add the tilapia and sear for 3 minutes per side. Using a slotted spatula, transfer to a plate and keep warm.

5. To the skillet, add the kale, bell pepper, and remaining 1½ tablespoons of taco seasoning. Cook, stirring occasionally, for 3 to 5 minutes, or until the veggies are tender. Remove from the heat.

6. Plate the tilapia over the grits and top with the colorful veggies for a restaurant-worthy presentation that keeps all the flavors together in one well-rounded bite.

FOIL-WRAPPED TUSCAN HADDOCK

SERVES 4 | **PREP TIME:** 5 MINUTES | **COOK TIME:** 15 MINUTES

30-MINUTE MEAL | **LEFTOVER-FRIENDLY** | **GLUTEN-FREE** | **NUT-FREE**

Baking fillets in aluminum foil is one of the easiest, most convenient ways to prepare fish. The result is a moist and tender fish with well-infused flavor from all the veggies and seasoning. Simply serve over rice, and you've got a complete meal. You can also serve the fish and veggies over ½ cup of cooked angel hair pasta for a slightly different texture.

Nonstick cooking spray, for coating

2 (6-ounce) haddock fillets, rinsed and patted dry

2 teaspoons Tuscan seasoning

4 teaspoons olive oil, divided

1 medium zucchini, thinly sliced

2 cups frozen tricolor bell pepper strips

2 cups frozen brown rice

PER SERVING (¼ OF THE RECIPE): Calories: 280; Fat: 10g; Carbohydrates: 24g; Protein: 21g; Fiber: 5g; Sodium: 260mg; Iron: 2mg

1. Preheat the oven to 400°F. Lay out 8 large sheets of aluminum foil and lightly coat 4 of them with cooking spray.

2. Divide each fillet into 2 equal portions. Place 1 haddock portion on each piece of coated foil.

3. Top each with ½ teaspoon of Tuscan seasoning and 1 teaspoon of olive oil.

4. Layer equal amounts of zucchini and bell pepper on each haddock portion.

5. Place the remaining sheets of foil over each and crimp to seal the packets tightly. Transfer to a baking sheet.

6. Transfer the baking sheet to the oven and bake for 10 to 15 minutes, or until the haddock flakes easily with a fork. Remove from the oven.

7. Meanwhile, prepare the rice in the microwave according to the package instructions, usually about 3 minutes.

8. Serve the fish and veggies, juice and all, over the brown rice.

HADDOCK WITH CREAMY YOGURT MAYONNAISE

SERVES 4 | PREP TIME: 10 MINUTES **| COOK TIME:** 20 MINUTES

30-MINUTE MEAL | LEFTOVER-FRIENDLY | GLUTEN-FREE | NUT-FREE

The yogurt mayonnaise that pairs with haddock in this dish has all the creaminess of a mayonnaise but without all the fat. Adding just a couple tablespoons of mayonnaise to a base of seasoned yogurt makes a blend perfectly suited for coating your fish to get a moist and flavorful result.

Nonstick cooking spray, for coating

½ cup plain low-fat Greek yogurt

2 tablespoons low-fat mayonnaise or 1½ tablespoons olive oil

1 teaspoon honey

1 teaspoon Dijon mustard

¼ teaspoon sea salt

2 (6-ounce) haddock fillets, rinsed and patted dry

4 teaspoons finely chopped chives or scallions, green parts only

Grated zest and juice of 1 medium lemon

2 tablespoons olive oil, divided

2 cups frozen brown rice

4 cups arugula

1. Preheat the oven to 375°F. Line a rimmed baking sheet or a 9-by-9-inch baking dish with aluminum foil. Coat with cooking spray.

2. In a small bowl, thoroughly combine the yogurt, mayonnaise, honey, mustard, and salt.

3. Put the haddock on the prepared baking sheet. Spread the yogurt mixture evenly over each fillet to thoroughly coat.

4. Top with the chives and lemon zest. Drizzle on 1 tablespoon of olive oil.

5. Transfer the baking sheet to the oven and bake for 15 to 20 minutes, or until the haddock flakes easily with a fork. There will be some juices from the fish mixed with the melting yogurt sauce. Remove from the oven.

6. Meanwhile, prepare the rice in the microwave according to the package instructions, usually 3 to 5 minutes.

7. In a medium bowl, toss the arugula with the lemon juice and remaining 1 tablespoon of olive oil.

8. Serve the haddock over the seasoned arugula with the brown rice on the side. Store leftovers in separate tightly sealed containers for 2 to 3 days.

SUBSTITUTION TIP: You can easily swap out haddock for cod—they are both mild white fish.

PER SERVING (1 BOWL): Calories: 260; Fat: 10g; Carbohydrates: 22g; Protein: 20g; Fiber: 2g; Sodium: 436mg; Iron: 1mg

TAHINI ROASTED SALMON WITH WARM KALE SALAD

SERVES 4 | **PREP TIME:** 10 MINUTES | **COOK TIME:** 20 MINUTES

30-MINUTE MEAL | **LEFTOVER-FRIENDLY** | **NUT-FREE**

There are so many ways to flavor salmon for delicious roasted fillets. Having dressings prepared ahead of time makes it a breeze. Choose your dressing, slather it on the raw fillets, and roast to tender perfection. I use turmeric-tahini dressing here, which adds a sweet, tangy, slightly earthy glaze.

Nonstick cooking spray, for coating

2 (6-ounce) salmon fillets, rinsed and patted dry

½ cup Turmeric-Tahini Dressing (page 195)

8 cups water

1⅓ teaspoons sea salt, plus ⅛ teaspoon

4 cups chopped lacinato kale

1 tablespoon olive oil

3 garlic cloves, minced

1 cup canned chickpeas, drained and rinsed

PER SERVING (¼ OF THE RECIPE): Calories: 260; Fat: 13g; Carbohydrates: 13g; Protein: 22g; Fiber: 4g; Sodium: 267mg; Iron: 2mg

1. Preheat the oven to 425°F. Line a rimmed baking sheet or a 9-by-9-inch baking dish with aluminum foil. Coat with cooking spray.

2. Put the salmon on the prepared baking sheet. Coat evenly with the dressing.

3. Transfer the baking sheet to the oven and bake for 15 to 20 minutes, or until the flesh flakes easily with a fork. Remove from the oven.

4. Meanwhile, prepare the kale. In a large pot, combine the water and 1⅓ teaspoons of salt. Bring to a boil over high heat. Fill a bowl with cold water.

5. Add the kale to the pot and cook for 1 to 2 minutes, or until wilted and bright green. Remove from the heat. Immediately drain the kale and place it in the bowl of cold water. Once cool, drain the kale again, then use a salad spinner or towel to wring out excess water.

6. In a large, high-sided pan or soup pot, heat the olive oil over medium-high heat for 1 minute, or until shimmering.

7. Add the garlic and remaining ⅛ teaspoon of salt. Cook for 1 to 2 minutes, or until the garlic has lightly browned. Remove from the pan.

8. Add the kale and chickpeas to the pan. Cook, stirring occasionally, for about 5 minutes, or until the kale and chickpeas are warm. Remove from the heat.

9. Mix in the toasted garlic.

10. Serve the salmon over the kale. Refrigerate leftovers in an airtight container for 2 to 3 days.

VARIATION TIP: For an equally tasty variation, swap out the chickpeas for an equal amount of cannellini beans and season with Italian spices in addition to the toasted garlic.

BAKED SALMON WITH CREAMY CILANTRO DRESSING

SERVES 4 | **PREP TIME:** 10 MINUTES | **COOK TIME:** 20 MINUTES

30-MINUTE MEAL | **ONE POT/PAN** | **LEFTOVER-FRIENDLY** | **GLUTEN-FREE** | **NUT-FREE**

Cook the salmon first, then dress it with creamy cilantro dressing to get the optimal freshness of the cilantro infused in the tangy yogurt base. You'll kill two birds with one stone by roasting the salmon with the broccoli.

Nonstick cooking spray, for coating

½ cup Creamy Cilantro Dressing (page 194)

2 (6-ounce) salmon fillets, rinsed and patted dry

4 cups small broccoli florets

6 teaspoons olive oil, divided

1 recipe Sweet Potato Medallions (page 203)

PER SERVING (1 BOWL):
Calories: 310; Fat: 16g; Carbohydrates: 21g; Protein: 23g; Fiber: 5g; Sodium: 310mg; Iron: 2mg

1. Preheat the oven to 425°F. Line a rimmed baking sheet or a 9-by-9-inch baking dish with aluminum foil. Coat with cooking spray.

2. Place the salmon fillets in the center of the prepared baking sheet with the broccoli florets scattered around them. Drizzle 2 teaspoons of oil onto each fillet, then distribute the remaining 2 teaspoons of oil over the broccoli.

3. Transfer the baking sheet to the oven and bake for 15 to 20 minutes, or until the salmon flakes easily with a fork and the broccoli is tender. If the broccoli is not tender enough after this time, remove the salmon, and continue to cook the broccoli for 5 minutes, or until slightly crisp and easily pierced with a fork. Remove from the oven.

4. Serve the salmon over the sweet potatoes with the broccoli on the side. Refrigerate leftovers in an airtight container for 2 to 3 days.

VARIATION TIP: For a simpler sweet potato option, cut 2 medium sweet potatoes into ¼-inch rounds. Place them in a microwave-safe dish with ¼ cup of water. Cover and microwave for 5 minutes, or until tender. Drain and season with ⅛ teaspoon sea salt.

TERIYAKI SALMON BOWLS

SERVES 4 | PREP TIME: 10 MINUTES | COOK TIME: 15 MINUTES

30-MINUTE MEAL | LEFTOVER-FRIENDLY | NUT-FREE

Don't have any salmon already prepared? No worries. This recipe is easy to make from scratch, and you can save any leftover fish for use in other weekday lunch bowls. It's great for macro bowls or bulking up leafy green salads with some added protein.

Nonstick cooking spray, for coating

2 (6-ounce) salmon fillets, rinsed and patted dry

¾ cup Date-Sweetened Teriyaki Sauce (page 190)

4 cups fresh baby spinach

1 cup shelled edamame

1 cup grated carrots

1 medium ripe avocado, pitted, peeled, and diced

4 scallions, chopped, green parts only

4 teaspoons toasted sesame seeds or toasted flaxseed (optional)

PER SERVING (1 BOWL):
Calories: 333; Fat: 13g; Carbohydrates: 29g; Protein: 30g; Fiber: 11g; Sodium: 687mg; Iron: 8mg

1. Preheat the oven to 425°F. Line a rimmed baking sheet or a 9-by-9-inch baking dish with aluminum foil, then coat the foil with cooking spray.

2. Put the salmon fillets on the prepared baking sheet and coat well with an even layer of teriyaki sauce.

3. Transfer the baking sheet to the oven and bake for 15 minutes, or until the salmon flakes easily with a fork. Remove from the oven.

4. Meanwhile, steam the spinach. Fill a medium pot with a few inches of water and insert a steamer basket. Bring to a boil over medium heat.

5. Put the spinach in the steamer. Cover the pot and cook for about 3 minutes, or until the spinach is just wilted. Remove from the heat.

6. Layer 4 bowls evenly with the spinach, edamame, carrots, salmon, and avocado.

7. Garnish with the scallions and toasted sesame seeds (if using). Refrigerate leftover salmon in an airtight container for 2 to 3 days.

INGREDIENT TIP: For a marinated option, put the salmon fillets in a resealable bag with the teriyaki sauce and refrigerate for 3 hours. Then remove from the bag and follow the recipe as written.

AVOCADO-DILL POACHED SALMON

SERVES 4 | **PREP TIME:** 10 MINUTES | **COOK TIME:** 10 MINUTES

30-MINUTE MEAL | **LEFTOVER-FRIENDLY** | **NUT-FREE**

You'll notice that this recipe calls for skin-on salmon—the skin helps hold the fillets together while they poach. To prevent waste, prepare the Avocado-Dill Dressing (page 196) first, if not already on hand, and add the juiced lemons to the poaching liquid.

1½ cups low-sodium vegetable broth

1½ cups water

¼ cup dry white wine

1 lemon, thinly sliced (see headnote)

2 teaspoons coarsely chopped fresh dill, plus 2 dill sprigs

2 (6-ounce) skin-on salmon fillets, rinsed and patted dry

4 cups chopped romaine lettuce

4 medium vine-ripened tomatoes, sliced

½ medium cucumber, sliced

4 scallions, green parts only, chopped

2 tablespoons Avocado-Dill Dressing (page 196), plus ½ cup

2 sourdough bread slices, halved

Nonstick cooking spray, for coating

1. In a large skillet, combine the broth, water, wine, lemon (or lemon remains from the dressing preparation), and chopped dill. Bring to a boil over high heat.

2. Add the salmon. Reduce the heat to low. Cover the skillet and simmer for 10 minutes, or until the flesh flakes easily with a fork. Remove from the heat. Let cool.

3. Meanwhile, prepare the salad. In a large bowl, toss together the lettuce, tomatoes, cucumber, and scallions.

4. Coat evenly with 2 tablespoons of dressing.

5. Once the salmon has cooled, divide it into 4 portions.

6. Spread the remaining ½ cup of dressing onto the salmon (2 tablespoons per portion).

7. Garnish each portion with half of a dill sprig.

8. Toast the sourdough slices and coat them lightly with cooking spray. Serve the toast alongside the poached salmon and salad. (Or serve the poached salmon directly on the toast.)

9. Refrigerate salmon leftovers in an airtight container for 2 to 3 days. Leftover dressing will last for up to a week in the refrigerator.

INGREDIENT TIP: Like the Creamy Cilantro Dressing (page 194), Avocado-Dill Dressing adds delicious flavor to baked sweet potatoes or sweet potato medallions.

SUBSTITUTION TIP: If you don't have wine on hand (or cannot have alcohol), swap out the white wine for 2 tablespoons apple cider vinegar.

PER SERVING (¼ OF THE RECIPE): Calories: 320; Fat: 22g; Carbohydrates: 11g; Protein: 20g; Fiber: 4g; Sodium: 359mg; Iron: 2mg

SESAME SALMON PROTEIN BOWLS

SERVES 4 | **PREP TIME:** 10 MINUTES | **COOK TIME:** 20 MINUTES

30-MINUTE MEAL | **LEFTOVER-FRIENDLY** | **NUT-FREE**

This bowl includes two flavorful, healthy fats: salmon, which is rich in omega-3 fatty acids, and avocado, a great source of monounsaturated (healthy) fat. The sesame seed garnish adds a light, toasty, tasty crunch. The pickled radish takes three days to cure, so make a batch well ahead of when you want to eat this dish.

Nonstick cooking spray, for coating

2 (6-ounce) salmon fillets, rinsed and patted dry

½ cup Sesame Dressing (page 193)

2 cups sliced carrots

2 cups sliced zucchini

1⅓ cups frozen brown rice

1 medium, ripe avocado, pitted, peeled, and diced

4 teaspoons toasted sesame seeds

4 tablespoons sliced Ginger Pickled Radish (page 200)

PER SERVING (1 BOWL):
Calories: 446; Fat: 25g; Protein: 23g; Carbohydrates: 35g; Fiber: 8g; Sodium: 242mg; Iron: 2mg

1. Preheat the oven to 425°F. Line a rimmed baking sheet or a 9-by-13-inch baking dish with aluminum foil. Coat with cooking spray.

2. Put the salmon on the prepared baking sheet and coat the tops of the fillets evenly with the dressing.

3. Transfer the baking sheet to the oven and bake for 15 to 20 minutes, or until the flesh flakes easily with a fork. Remove from the oven.

4. Meanwhile, fill a large pot with a few inches of water and insert a steamer basket.

5. Put the carrots in the basket and bring the water to a boil over high heat. Cover the pot and steam for 5 minutes, or until the carrots begin to soften.

6. Add the zucchini, cover, and steam for another 5 minutes, or until all the veggies are soft. Remove from the heat.

7. Prepare the rice in the microwave according to the package instructions, usually about 3 minutes. Divide evenly among 4 bowls.

8. Layer each bowl with the zucchini and carrots.

9. Halve the salmon fillets and place a piece in each bowl.

10. Garnish each bowl with 2 tablespoons of chopped avocado, 1 teaspoon of sesame seeds, and 1 tablespoon of pickled radish. Serve.

TECHNICAL TIP: The more evenly the fish fillets are cut, the more evenly they will cook. Look for fillets that have the same thickness all around so one part doesn't come out drier than another.

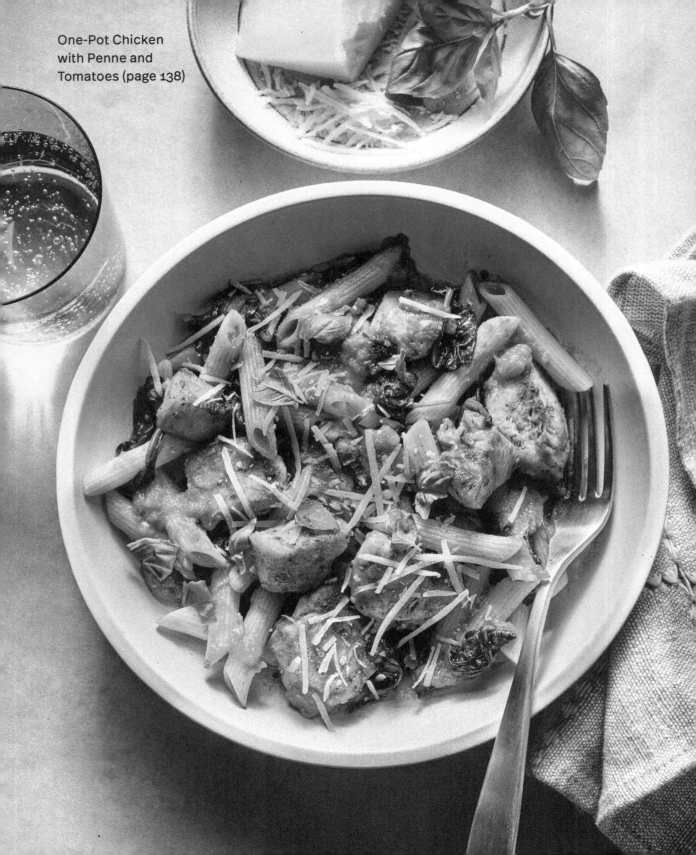

One-Pot Chicken
with Penne and
Tomatoes (page 138)

CHAPTER 7

POULTRY

Sesame Chicken Chopped Salad **120**

Cashew Chicken **121**

Herbed Chicken with Couscous and Spinach **122**

Fiesta Chicken Macro Bowls **124**

Pineapple Chicken **126**

Panko-Crusted Chicken with Dipping Sauce Trio **128**

Simple Baked Chicken with Potato and Green Bean Salad **130**

Dijon Roasted Chicken with Grits **132**

Teriyaki Chicken with Kale Salad and Sweet Potato Medallions **134**

Chicken Parmesan **136**

One-Pot Chicken with Penne and Tomatoes **138**

One-Pot Pasta with Ground Turkey and Mushroom Sauce **139**

Turkey Burgers with Creamy Cilantro Dressing **140**

Turkey, Apple, and Cranberry Meatballs **142**

Italian Wedding Soup **144**

Barbecue Turkey Bowls **146**

SESAME CHICKEN CHOPPED SALAD

SERVES 4 | PREP TIME: 10 MINUTES
30-MINUTE MEAL | ONE POT/PAN

Edamame adds plant protein to this salad, which means you can use less chicken and still have plenty of protein. It is rich in fiber, antioxidants, and vitamin K (a vitamin key to helping heal wounds and prevent excessive bleeding). Save yourself chopping time by using pre-shredded cabbage (or coleslaw mix) and shredded carrots. Shredding cabbage is easy if you've got a food processor, but precut veggies can be quite convenient.

½ recipe Simple Baked Chicken with Potato and Green Bean Salad (page 130), chicken only

2½ cups shredded cabbage

1 cup grated carrots

1 cup chopped romaine lettuce

½ cup shelled edamame

¼ cup sliced almonds

¼ cup chopped scallions, green parts only

½ cup Sesame Dressing (page 193)

½ cup Crispy Chickpeas (page 201)

1. Let the chicken cool for 5 to 10 minutes before cutting it into a ½-inch dice or strips.

2. In a large salad bowl, combine the cabbage, carrots, lettuce, edamame, almonds, and scallions.

3. Add the chicken and dressing. Toss well to coat.

4. Garnish with the chickpeas and serve.

VARIATION TIP: If you don't have the Crispy Chickpeas on hand, you can replace them with another ½ cup shelled edamame.

PER SERVING (¼ OF THE RECIPE): Calories: 321; Fat: 17g; Carbohydrates: 22g; Protein: 22g; Fiber: 7g; Sodium: 496mg; Iron: 2mg

CASHEW CHICKEN

SERVES 6 | PREP TIME: 10 MINUTES **| COOK TIME:** 10 TO 15 MINUTES
30-MINUTE MEAL | LEFTOVER-FRIENDLY

This cashew chicken takes little more than 20 minutes to make–using frozen veggies makes it simple and saves you time. With toasted cashews and the savory appeal of ginger, garlic, and soy in the teriyaki sauce, you'll have a delicious combo to serve over rice.

1½ tablespoons olive oil

5 (4-ounce) boneless, skinless chicken thighs, chopped into 1½-inch pieces

3 cups frozen tricolor bell pepper strips

3 cups frozen cut green beans

⅓ cup water

1 tablespoon cornstarch

⅓ cup Date-Sweetened Teriyaki Sauce (page 190)

1½ teaspoons white miso or low-sodium soy sauce

3 cups frozen brown rice

1 cup roasted unsalted cashews

⅓ cup chopped scallions, green parts only

PER SERVING (⅙ OF THE RECIPE): Calories: 466; Fat: 19g; Carbohydrates: 40g; Protein: 34g; Fiber: 8g; Sodium: 314mg; Iron: 4mg

1. In a medium skillet, heat the oil over medium-high heat for 1 minute, or until shimmering.

2. Carefully add the chicken and cook, stirring occasionally, for 5 minutes, or until lightly browned and thoroughly cooked. Using a slotted spoon or spatula, transfer to a plate.

3. Reduce the heat to medium. Add the bell pepper and green beans to the skillet.

4. Stir in the water and cornstarch.

5. Add the teriyaki sauce and miso. Mix well. Cook for 5 minutes, or until the veggies have warmed and the sauce has thickened.

6. Meanwhile, cook the rice according to the package instructions, usually about 3 minutes in the microwave.

7. Return the cooked chicken to the skillet. Add the cashews and cook for another minute, or until the dish is evenly warmed. Remove from the heat.

8. Serve the chicken and veggies over the rice.

9. Garnish with the scallions. Refrigerate leftovers in an airtight container for up to 3 days.

TECHNICAL TIP: Poultry scissors make it easy to chop the chicken. Additionally, a pair of plastic disposable gloves can be useful if you don't want to touch the chicken.

HERBED CHICKEN WITH COUSCOUS AND SPINACH

SERVES 4 | PREP TIME: 10 MINUTES **| COOK TIME:** 20 MINUTES

30-MINUTE MEAL | LEFTOVER-FRIENDLY | NUT-FREE

A quick panko mixture with a few common spices and a bit of sea salt gives your baked chicken an herbal quality that will complement the simply flavored couscous and fresh spinach of this recipe well.

Nonstick cooking spray, for coating the baking dish

⅓ cup panko bread crumbs

¾ teaspoon garlic powder, divided

¼ teaspoon dried basil

⅛ teaspoon dried thyme

¼ teaspoon sea salt, divided

2 tablespoons olive oil, divided

4 (4-ounce) boneless, skinless chicken breasts

2⅔ cups water

1⅓ cups dried couscous

4 cups baby spinach

¼ cup grated parmesan cheese

PER SERVING (¼ OF THE RECIPE): Calories: 531; Fat: 14g; Carbohydrates: 52g; Protein: 46g; Fiber: 4g; Sodium: 374mg; Iron: 2mg

1. Preheat the oven to 425°F. Lightly coat a 9-by-13-inch baking dish with cooking spray.

2. In a small bowl, combine the bread crumbs, ½ teaspoon of garlic powder, the basil, thyme, and ⅛ teaspoon of salt.

3. Use 1 tablespoon of olive oil to coat both sides of each chicken breast. Season with the remaining ⅛ teaspoon of salt.

4. Put the chicken in the baking dish and evenly distribute the panko-herb mixture over the chicken. Drizzle with the remaining 1 tablespoon of olive oil.

5. Transfer the baking dish to the oven and bake for 20 minutes, or until the chicken is no longer pink inside and reaches an internal temperature of 160°F. Remove from the oven. Let rest for about 5 minutes before serving, or until the internal temperature reaches 165°F.

6. While the chicken is baking, in a medium soup pot, combine the water and remaining ¼ teaspoon of garlic powder. Bring to a boil over medium heat.

7. Stir in the couscous, then turn off the heat. Place a steamer basket in the pot.

8. Put the spinach in the steamer basket. Cover the pot and steam for 6 minutes, or until all the water has been absorbed into the couscous and the spinach has wilted. Remove from the heat.

9. Plate the chicken over the spinach with the couscous on the side. Serve. Refrigerate leftovers in separate airtight containers: couscous for up to 2 days; herbed chicken for up to 4 days.

TECHNICAL TIP: Letting the chicken rest before serving keeps it tender by preventing the juices from escaping.

FIESTA CHICKEN MACRO BOWLS

SERVES 4 | PREP TIME: 15 MINUTES | **COOK TIME:** 10 MINUTES
30-MINUTE MEAL | LEFTOVER-FRIENDLY | GLUTEN-FREE | NUT-FREE

With zesty chicken, black beans, corn, and seasoned kale, this chicken bowl is full of flavor. Creamy cilantro dressing is an optional way to brighten the dish with freshness and tang; however, the bowl is already delicious on its own.

2 tablespoons olive oil, divided

3 (4-ounce) boneless, skinless chicken breasts, cut into 1-inch chunks

1 tablespoon DIY Taco Seasoning (page 198)

1 (14½-ounce) can low-sodium black beans, drained and rinsed

2 tablespoons chopped scallions, green parts only

¼ cup low-sodium chicken broth

2 cups frozen corn

6 cups chopped stemmed kale

⅛ teaspoon sea salt

Juice of 1 lemon

1 medium, ripe avocado, peeled and sliced

¼ cup Creamy Cilantro Dressing (page 194), divided (optional)

1. In a medium skillet, heat 1 tablespoon of oil over medium heat for 1 minute, or until shimmering.

2. Add the chicken and taco seasoning. Using a spatula, mix well. Cook, stirring, for 5 minutes, or until no longer pink inside. Remove to a plate.

3. To the skillet, add the beans, scallions, and broth. Stir for 1 minute, or until all the liquid has been absorbed.

4. Reduce the heat to medium-low. Push the veggies to one side of the skillet. Add the corn and cook for 1 minute, or until warmed, then mix with the veggies. Remove from the heat. Cover the skillet.

5. In a large bowl, combine the kale, salt, remaining 1 tablespoon of oil, and the lemon juice. Using clean hands, massage the kale until reduced to about half the size.

6. Divide the chicken, beans, corn, and kale mixture among 4 bowls.

7. Garnish with the avocado.

8. For extra flavor, drizzle each bowl with 1 tablespoon of cilantro dressing (if using). Refrigerate leftovers in an airtight container for up to 4 days. Wrap any remaining avocado tightly with plastic wrap, keeping the pit intact, and eat within 2 days.

VARIATION TIP: Another tangy way to enhance the dish is to swap out the creamy cilantro dressing for 2 tablespoons plain low-fat Greek yogurt.

PER SERVING (¼ OF THE RECIPE): Calories: 495; Fat: 22g; Carbohydrates: 40g; Protein: 38g; Fiber: 13g; Sodium: 568mg; Iron: 4mg

PINEAPPLE CHICKEN

SERVES 4 | PREP TIME: 10 MINUTES **| COOK TIME:** 20 TO 25 MINUTES

LEFTOVER-FRIENDLY | NUT-FREE

This is a wonderful variation of simple baked chicken, with honey-soy glaze and crushed pineapple added toward the end of the cooking process. Basting is key to keeping those tasty juices from escaping the chicken (and you'll still have some extra jus to flavor your rice).

Nonstick cooking spray, for coating the baking dish

¼ cup honey

2 tablespoons low-sodium soy sauce

4 (4-ounce) boneless, skinless chicken thighs

1 tablespoon olive oil

⅛ teaspoon sea salt

½ cup canned crushed pineapple, drained

¼ cup chopped scallions, green parts only

2 cups frozen short-grain brown rice

2 cups frozen cut green beans

¼ cup water

PER SERVING (¼ OF THE RECIPE): Calories: 413; Fat: 11g; Carbohydrates: 44g; Protein: 36g; Fiber: 4g; Sodium: 501mg; Iron: 3mg

1. Preheat the oven to 425°F. Lightly coat a 9-by-13-inch baking dish with cooking spray.

2. To make the glaze, in a small bowl, whisk together the honey and soy sauce until thick and viscous.

3. Coat both sides of each chicken thigh with the olive oil. Season with the salt.

4. Put the chicken in the prepared baking dish. Seal with aluminum foil.

5. Transfer the baking dish to the oven and bake for 15 minutes.

6. Brush the chicken with the glaze, then reseal the baking dish with the foil. Return the baking dish to the oven and roast, basting halfway through, for another 5 minutes, or until the internal temperature of the chicken reaches 160°F. Remove from the oven. Reserve the extra juice for flavoring the rice.

7. Set the oven to broil.

8. Top the chicken with the pineapple and scallions.

9. Return the baking dish to the oven and broil for 1 minute, or until the topping has warmed. Remove from the oven. Let the chicken cool for 5 minutes, or until the internal temperature reaches 165°F.

10. While the chicken is baking, prepare the rice in the microwave according to the package instructions, usually about 3 minutes.

11. In a microwave-safe bowl, combine the green beans and water. Cover and microwave for 4 minutes, or until tender. Drain any excess water.

12. Serve the pineapple chicken with the green beans and rice. Use extra juices from the chicken to flavor the rice. Refrigerate leftovers in an airtight container for up to 3 days.

PANKO-CRUSTED CHICKEN WITH DIPPING SAUCE TRIO

SERVES 4 | **PREP TIME:** 10 MINUTES | **COOK TIME:** 15 MINUTES

30-MINUTE MEAL | **LEFTOVER-FRIENDLY** | **NUT-FREE**

You can choose any of the staple creamy dressings in this book for your dipping trio, but I've provided one of my absolute favorites—creamy cilantro dressing—plus two simple combos you can make in a jiffy. The crispy chicken is absolutely delicious dunked in these sauces. You and your kids will love it.

For the dipping trio

½ cup Creamy Cilantro Dressing (page 194) or Date-Sweetened Barbecue Sauce (page 191)

Garlic-Dijon Sauce:

¼ cup low-fat mayonnaise

2 teaspoons Dijon mustard

1 garlic clove, minced

Thousand Island Sauce:

¼ cup ketchup

2 tablespoons low-fat mayonnaise

2 tablespoons plain low-fat Greek yogurt

2 tablespoons pickle relish

For the chicken

¼ cup all-purpose flour

1 medium egg, beaten

¾ cup panko bread crumbs

4 (4-ounce) boneless, skinless chicken breasts, cut into strips

2½ tablespoons olive oil

4 cups broccoli florets

¼ cup water

To make the dipping trio

1. If not already prepared, make the cilantro dressing or barbecue sauce (or any other dressing from chapter 10).
2. To make the garlic-Dijon sauce, in a small bowl, whisk together the mayonnaise, mustard, and garlic.
3. To make the thousand island sauce, in a small bowl, whisk together the ketchup, mayonnaise, yogurt, and pickle relish.

To make the chicken

4. Set up a breading station. Put the flour, egg, and bread crumbs in 3 separate small bowls.
5. Dredge each piece of chicken in the flour, then dip in the egg, and lastly coat it in the bread crumbs. Place on a large plate.
6. In a large skillet, heat the oil over medium-high heat for 1 minute, or until shimmering.
7. Reduce the heat to medium. Add the chicken and cook for 3 to 4 minutes per side, or until golden, crisp, and no longer pink inside. Remove from the heat. Let rest for 5 to 10 minutes, or until the internal temperature reaches 165°F.
8. In a microwave-safe bowl, combine the broccoli and water. Cover and microwave for 4 minutes, or until tender. Drain any excess water.
9. Serve the chicken with the 3 dipping sauces and the broccoli on the side. Refrigerate leftovers in an airtight container for up to 3 days.

PER SERVING (¼ OF THE RECIPE, INCLUDES PARMESAN):
Calories: 478; Fat: 23g; Carbohydrates: 34g; Protein: 36g; Fiber: 4g; Sodium: 678mg; Iron: 2mg

SIMPLE BAKED CHICKEN WITH POTATO AND GREEN BEAN SALAD

SERVES 6 | PREP TIME: 10 MINUTES **| COOK TIME:** 35 MINUTES

LEFTOVER-FRIENDLY | NUT-FREE

Tender and moist, this chicken is so versatile. Use it in entrées, salads, burritos—you name it!

For the chicken

Nonstick cooking spray, for coating the baking dish

6 (4-ounce) boneless, skinless chicken breasts

2 tablespoons olive oil

⅛ teaspoon sea salt

¼ teaspoon lemon pepper seasoning

For the salad

5 medium red potatoes

3 cups frozen cut green beans

¼ cup water

1 tablespoon olive oil

⅛ teaspoon sea salt

1½ teaspoons Dijon mustard or white miso

3 tablespoons chopped scallions, green parts only

To make the chicken

1. Preheat the oven to 425°F. Lightly coat a 9-by-13-inch baking dish with cooking spray.

2. Put the chicken in a large plastic bag and seal tightly. Lay the bag flat on a cutting board so the chicken is in one layer. Using the flat side of a meat mallet or the bottom of a can, pound the chicken evenly for 1 to 2 minutes, or until its thickness is reduced by half.

3. Add the oil, salt, and lemon pepper seasoning to the bag with the chicken. Shake vigorously to coat thoroughly. Transfer the chicken to the prepared baking dish. Seal with aluminum foil.

4. Transfer the baking dish to the oven and bake the chicken for 20 to 25 minutes, or until the internal temperature reaches 160°F and the juices run clear. Remove from the oven. Let cool for 5 minutes, or until the internal temperature of the chicken reaches 165°F.

To make the salad

5. While the chicken is baking, put the potatoes in a medium pot and cover them with water. Cook over medium-high heat for 30 minutes, or until the potatoes are fork-tender. Remove from the heat. Drain and let cool for 5 minutes.

6. Once the potatoes have cooled, chop them into 1½-inch chunks (you can leave the skin on).

7. In a medium microwave-safe bowl, combine the green beans and water. Cover and microwave for 4 minutes, or until tender. Drain.

8. To the green beans, add the potatoes, oil, salt, mustard, and scallions. Toss to combine.

9. Serve the chicken with the potato and green bean salad.

VARIATION TIP: To make this a baked curry chicken, use sweet potatoes instead of red potatoes and season with ¼ teaspoon of curry powder instead of the mustard. You can also replace the lemon pepper seasoning with ¼ teaspoon of curry powder.

PER SERVING (⅙ OF THE RECIPE): Calories: 404; Fat: 14g; Carbohydrates: 34g; Protein: 35g; Fiber: 6g; Sodium: 270mg; Iron: 5mg

DIJON ROASTED CHICKEN WITH GRITS

SERVES 4 | **PREP TIME:** 10 MINUTES | **COOK TIME:** 20 MINUTES

30-MINUTE MEAL | **LEFTOVER-FRIENDLY** | **NUT-FREE**

Cream of mushroom soup is the basis of the Dijon-flavored sauce in this chicken dish. With just a bit of turmeric, it takes on a golden yellow hue. The tang of the mustard chicken complements the creamy parmesan grits.

Nonstick cooking spray, for coating the baking dish

1 cup low-sodium cream of mushroom soup

2 teaspoons Dijon mustard

¼ teaspoon ground turmeric

1 tablespoon olive oil, plus 1 teaspoon

4 (4-ounce) boneless, skinless chicken breasts

⅛ teaspoon sea salt

4 teaspoons capers

4 parsley sprigs

1 cup instant grits

2¼ cups water, divided

¼ cup grated parmesan cheese

2 cups frozen green beans

PER SERVING (¼ OF THE RECIPE): Calories: 351; Fat: 13g; Carbohydrates: 19g; Protein: 40g; Fiber: 3g; Sodium: 762mg; Iron: 7mg

1. Preheat the oven to 425°F. Lightly coat a 9-by-13-inch baking dish with cooking spray.

2. In a medium bowl, combine the cream of mushroom soup, mustard, and turmeric.

3. Use 1 tablespoon of olive oil to coat both sides of each chicken breast. Season with the salt.

4. Put the chicken in the prepared baking dish. Evenly smother with the soup mixture.

5. Transfer the baking dish to the oven and bake for 20 minutes, or until the internal temperature reaches 160°F. Remove from the oven. Let the chicken rest for 5 to 10 minutes, or until the internal temperature reaches 165°F.

6. Garnish with the capers and parsley.

7. While the chicken is baking, prepare the grits. In a medium soup pot, combine the grits and 2 cups of water. Bring to a boil over medium heat. Cook for 6 minutes, or until the grits are smooth and creamy. Remove from the heat. Season with the remaining 1 teaspoon of olive oil.

8. Top the grits with the cheese.

9. While the grits are cooking, prepare the green beans. In a microwave-safe bowl, combine the green beans and remaining ¼ cup of water. Cover and microwave for 4 minutes, or until the beans have warmed through. Drain any excess water.

10. Serve the chicken over the grits with the green beans on the side, pouring any remaining sauce over the grits. Refrigerate leftovers in separate airtight containers: chicken for up to 4 days; grits and green beans for up to 1 week.

VARIATION TIP: Swap out the cream of mushroom soup for cream of broccoli soup for a slightly different flavor.

TERIYAKI CHICKEN WITH KALE SALAD AND SWEET POTATO MEDALLIONS

SERVES 4 | PREP TIME: 10 MINUTES | **COOK TIME:** 25 MINUTES

LEFTOVER-FRIENDLY | NUT-FREE

This roasted chicken is delightfully dressed with date-sweetened teriyaki sauce, bell pepper, and scallions. In keeping with the Asian-inspired theme, the kale is seasoned with garlic and soy sauce. Served with roasted sweet potato medallions, this makes for tasty, colorful meal.

Nonstick cooking spray, for coating the baking dish

2½ tablespoons olive oil, divided

4 (4-ounce) bone-in, skinless chicken thighs

⅛ teaspoon sea salt

¾ cup Date-Sweetened Teriyaki Sauce (page 190)

1 large red bell pepper, cored and cut into strips

¼ cup chopped scallions, green parts only

6 cups chopped stemmed kale

1 teaspoon minced garlic

¼ teaspoon low-sodium soy sauce

1 recipe Sweet Potato Medallions (page 203)

1. Preheat the oven to 425°F. Lightly coat a 9-by-13-inch baking dish with cooking spray.

2. Use 2 tablespoons of olive oil to coat both sides of each chicken thigh. Season with the salt.

3. Put the chicken in the prepared baking dish. Cover with the teriyaki sauce to evenly coat.

4. Top with the bell pepper and scallions.

5. Transfer the baking dish to the oven and bake the chicken for 20 to 25 minutes, or until the internal temperature reaches 160°F and the juices run clear. Remove from the oven. Let the chicken cool for 5 minutes, or until the internal temperature reaches 165°F.

6. While the chicken is baking, make the salad. Put the kale, remaining ½ tablespoon of olive oil, the garlic, and soy sauce in a medium bowl. Using clean hands, massage the kale for about 1 minute, or until the volume of kale pieces is reduced by half.

7. Serve the chicken with the salad and sweet potatoes on the side. Refrigerate leftovers in an airtight container for up to 3 days.

INGREDIENT TIP: You can buy packaged pre-chopped, triple-rinsed kale to save yourself chopping time.

PER SERVING (¼ OF THE RECIPE): Calories: 386; Fat: 18g; Carbohydrates: 17g; Protein: 39g; Fiber: 4g; Sodium: 654mg; Iron: 3mg

CHICKEN PARMESAN

SERVES 6 | PREP TIME: 10 MINUTES | **COOK TIME:** 15 MINUTES

30-MINUTE MEAL | LEFTOVER-FRIENDLY | NUT-FREE

From skillet to oven, this dish can be on the table in less than 30 minutes, which is great for busy nights. The panko-crusted chicken is golden perfection, topped with a generous portion of marinara sauce and some cheese. Chicken parmesan is a simple, tasty meal that kids and adults are sure to love.

Nonstick cooking spray, for coating the baking dish

6 tablespoons all-purpose flour

2 medium eggs, beaten

¾ cup panko bread crumbs

6 (4-ounce) boneless, skinless chicken breast

3 tablespoons olive oil

1½ cups marinara sauce

¾ cup grated parmesan cheese

12 small fresh basil leaves

3 cups frozen green beans

¼ cup water

PER SERVING (⅙ OF THE RECIPE): Calories: 394; Fat: 16g; Carbohydrates: 27g; Protein: 35g; Fiber: 4g; Sodium: 545mg; Iron: 2mg

1. Preheat the oven to 425°F. Lightly coat a 9-by-13-inch baking dish with cooking spray.

2. Set up 3 small bowls: one with the flour, one with the eggs, and one with the bread crumbs.

3. Using tongs, dredge each piece of chicken in the flour, dip it in the eggs, and then coat it in the bread crumbs. Set on a plate.

4. In a large, oven-safe skillet, heat the olive oil over medium heat for 1 minute, or until shimmering.

5. Carefully place the coated chicken in the hot skillet. Cook for 3 to 4 minutes per side, or until golden brown with an internal temperature of 160°F. Remove from the heat.

6. Pour the marinara over the chicken in the skillet, then top with the cheese.

7. Transfer the skillet to the oven; bake for 5 minutes, or until the cheese has melted and the sauce is bubbly. Remove the skillet from the oven (don't forget to wear an oven mitt!). Let the chicken cool for 5 minutes, or until the internal temperature reaches 165°F.

8. Garnish each piece of chicken with some fresh basil.

9. Meanwhile, in a microwave-safe bowl, combine the green beans and water. Cover and microwave for 4 minutes, or until tender. Drain any excess water.

10. Serve the chicken parmesan hot with the green beans on the side. Refrigerate leftovers in an airtight container for up to 4 days.

SUBSTITUTION TIP: Although parmesan is pretty standard for this dish, you can use grated cheddar or mozzarella instead.

ONE-POT CHICKEN WITH PENNE AND TOMATOES

SERVES 6 | **PREP TIME:** 10 MINUTES | **COOK TIME:** 20 MINUTES

30-MINUTE MEAL | **ONE-POT/PAN** | **LEFTOVER-FRIENDLY** | **NUT-FREE**

When I discovered I could cook my pasta and "meat" sauce together in one vessel, what a time-saver it was. And not having to drain hot water—even better. To get the utmost flavor, I cooked the seasoned chicken first before adding the remaining ingredients to the same skillet.

1½ tablespoons olive oil

5 (4-ounce) boneless, skinless chicken breasts, cut into 1-inch pieces

1½ tablespoons DIY Taco Seasoning (page 198)

3 garlic cloves, minced

12 ounces penne pasta

3 cups low-sodium marinara sauce

4½ cups water

6 cups baby spinach

¾ cup grated parmesan cheese (optional)

1. In a large, high-rimmed skillet, heat the oil over medium heat for 1 minute, or until shimmering.

2. Add the chicken, taco seasoning, and garlic. Cook, stirring, for 5 minutes, or until the chicken is no longer pink inside.

3. Add the penne, marinara, and water. Bring to a boil. Cook for 8 minutes, or until the penne is al dente.

4. Add the spinach. Cover the skillet and cook for 2 minutes, or until the spinach wilts. Remove from the heat.

5. Sprinkle with the cheese (if using) and serve. Refrigerate leftovers in an airtight container for up to 4 days.

PER SERVING (⅙ OF THE RECIPE, INCLUDES PARMESAN): Calories: 478; Fat: 14g; Carbohydrates: 52g; Protein: 34g; Fiber: 5g; Sodium: 553mg; Iron: 4mg

SUBSTITUTION TIP: If you don't have any taco seasoning prepared, you can replace it with ½ to 1 teaspoon Tuscan seasoning instead.

ONE-POT PASTA WITH GROUND TURKEY AND MUSHROOM SAUCE

SERVES 4 | PREP TIME: 10 MINUTES **| COOK TIME:** 20 MINUTES

30-MINUTE MEAL | ONE POT/PAN | LEFTOVER-FRIENDLY | NUT-FREE

This is a unique way to prepare a satisfying, tasty pasta dish without using several pans or utensils. Prepare the ground turkey first, add the veggies, and use the same pan to prepare the pasta for an all-in-one-pot meal.

2 tablespoons olive oil

8 ounces lean
   ground turkey

⅛ teaspoon sea salt

1 small yellow
   onion, chopped

4 cups small
   broccoli florets

½ teaspoon garlic
   powder, divided

⅛ teaspoon Italian
   seasoning

8 ounces flat egg noodles

4 cups water

1 cup low-sodium cream of
   mushroom soup

**PER SERVING (¼ OF THE
RECIPE):** Calories: 467;
Fat: 18g; Carbohydrates:
51g; Protein: 27g; Fiber: 5g;
Sodium: 272mg; Iron: 4mg

1. In a large, high-rimmed skillet, heat the oil over medium-high heat for 1 minute, or until shimmering.

2. Add the ground turkey and salt. Cook for 5 to 6 minutes, stirring often with a spatula to break the turkey into small pieces, for 5 to 6 minutes, or until the turkey is mostly browned.

3. Add the onion, broccoli, ¼ teaspoon of garlic powder, and the Italian seasoning.

4. Reduce the heat to medium. Cook, stirring occasionally, for 5 minutes, or until the onion is soft and the broccoli is tender-crisp.

5. Add the noodles, water, cream of mushroom soup, and remaining ¼ teaspoon of garlic powder. Bring to a boil. Cook for 9 minutes, or until the pasta is al dente. Remove from the heat. Serve warm. Refrigerate leftovers in an airtight container for up to 3 days.

VARIATION TIP: Swap out the broccoli for an equal amount of frozen green beans (no need to thaw before cooking).

TURKEY BURGERS WITH CREAMY CILANTRO DRESSING

SERVES 4 | **PREP TIME:** 10 MINUTES | **COOK TIME:** 20 MINUTES

30-MINUTE MEAL | **NUT-FREE**

Turkey burgers are tasty and convenient, but what you top your burger with can make all the difference when it comes to overall nutrition. Packed with bell pepper, crisp romaine, and tangy, versatile cilantro dressing, this is a delicious, well-rounded meal.

1 tablespoon olive oil

⅛ teaspoon sea salt

4 cups frozen tricolor bell pepper strips

12 ounces ground turkey

2 teaspoons low-sodium Worcestershire sauce

¼ teaspoon garlic powder

8 tablespoons Creamy Cilantro Dressing (page 194)

4 whole-wheat hamburger buns

8 large, crisp romaine lettuce leaves

PER SERVING (¼ OF THE RECIPE): Calories: 391; Fat: 17g; Carbohydrates: 34g; Protein: 24g; Fiber: 10g; Sodium: 478mg; Iron: 4mg

1. In a large skillet, heat the oil and salt over medium-high heat for 1 minute, or until the oil is shimmering.
2. Add the bell pepper and cook, stirring occasionally, for 3 minutes, or until browned on the edges.
3. Reduce the heat to low. Cover the skillet and cook for 5 minutes, or until the bell pepper is tender. Remove from the heat. Transfer to a plate.
4. Meanwhile, in a bowl, season the ground turkey with the Worcestershire sauce and garlic powder.
5. Using clean hands, form the turkey into 4 patties that are 3 inches in diameter.
6. Increase the heat to medium-high. Place two patties in the skillet. Cook for 6 minutes per side, or until browned and no longer pink inside. Remove from the heat. Repeat with the remaining patties.

7. Spread 2 tablespoons of dressing on both sides of each bun.
8. Layer each bun with the lettuce, a patty, and the bell pepper.

INGREDIENT TIP: For time-saving convenience, you can buy frozen turkey burger patties. Just be sure they are 100 percent turkey–nothing added.

VARIATION TIP: If you've got a batch of Ginger Pickled Radish (page 200) on hand, add 3 to 5 slices for a tangy punch (much like a dill pickle).

TURKEY, APPLE, AND CRANBERRY MEATBALLS

SERVES 4 | PREP TIME: 10 MINUTES **| COOK TIME:** 20 MINUTES

30-MINUTE MEAL

These unconventional meatballs are made with apples and cranberries for a savory-sweet combo.

8 ounces lean
  ground turkey

½ cup chopped Fuji apple

½ cup panko bread crumbs

¼ cup finely
  chopped walnuts

3 tablespoons
  dried cranberries,
  coarsely chopped

1 medium egg

2 teaspoons onion
  powder, divided

¼ teaspoon sea salt plus
  1 pinch, divided

2 medium sweet potatoes,
  thinly sliced

2 teaspoons olive oil, plus
  2 tablespoons

4 cups frozen green beans

½ cup water

3 tablespoons
  all-purpose flour

1 cup low-sodium
  chicken broth

⅛ teaspoon low-sodium
  Worcestershire sauce

Freshly ground
  black pepper

1. Preheat the oven to 400°F.

2. In a large bowl, using clean hands, mix together the ground turkey, apple, bread crumbs, walnuts, cranberries, egg, 1 teaspoon of onion powder, and ⅛ teaspoon of salt until well combined.

3. Roll the mixture into 1-inch balls. Place the meatballs on one side of a large baking sheet, and place the sweet potatoes on the other side, all in one flat layer. Drizzle 2 teaspoons of oil over the sweet potatoes. Sprinkle with ⅛ teaspoon of salt.

4. Transfer the baking sheet to the oven and bake for 15 to 20 minutes, or until the meatballs reach an internal temperature of 160°F and the sweet potatoes are al dente. Remove from the oven.

5. Meanwhile, in a microwave-safe dish, combine the green beans and water. Cover and microwave for 4 to 5 minutes, or until thoroughly warmed. Drain any excess water.

6.   While the beans are cooking, make the gravy. In a medium skillet or saucepan, whisk together the remaining 2 tablespoons of oil, the flour, and the remaining 1 teaspoon of onion powder over medium heat for about 1 minute, or until a roux (paste) forms.

7.   Slowly whisk in the broth for 2 to 3 minutes, or until the mixture thickens into a gravy. For a thicker gravy, use a little less broth (although the gravy will thicken as it sits). To thin it out, continue to heat and stir while adding 1 to 2 tablespoons of water at a time until you reach your desired consistency. Remove from the heat. Season with the remaining pinch of salt, the Worcestershire sauce, and black pepper.

8.   Drizzle the gravy over the meatballs and serve with the sweet potatoes and green beans on the side.

VARIATION TIP: Swap out the onion powder for an equal amount of diced fennel bulb and add a few tablespoons of finely chopped parsley to the meatball mixture.

PER SERVING (¼ OF THE RECIPE): Calories: 470; Fat: 22g; Carbohydrates: 47g; Protein: 24g; Fiber: 8g; Sodium: 293mg; Iron: 3mg

ITALIAN WEDDING SOUP

SERVES 4 | **PREP TIME:** 10 MINUTES | **COOK TIME:** 25 MINUTES
LEFTOVER-FRIENDLY | **NUT-FREE**

Italian wedding soup is traditional to southern Italy, and its name refers to the marriage of ingredients: namely meatballs (or sausage) and leafy greens. You'll find versions that include a combo of ground meats such as pork and beef, bitter greens such as escarole, and pearls of Italian pasta known as *acini de pepe*, likely named for their peppercorn size, shape, or both. This version of the soup uses ground turkey, spinach, and pearl couscous.

12 ounces lean ground turkey

⅓ cup grated parmesan cheese

⅓ cup panko bread crumbs

¼ cup chopped fresh cilantro or parsley

1 teaspoon Italian seasoning, divided

¼ teaspoon sea salt, divided

1 tablespoon olive oil, plus 1 teaspoon

1 small yellow onion, finely chopped

2 garlic cloves, minced

2¼ cups low-sodium chicken broth

2 cups water

1 cup dried pearl couscous

3 cups baby spinach

Juice of 1 lemon

1. In a large bowl, using clean hands, mix together the ground turkey, cheese, bread crumbs, parsley, ½ teaspoon of Italian seasoning, and ⅛ teaspoon of salt until well combined.

2. Shape the mixture into ¾-inch meatballs.

3. In a large stockpot, heat 1 tablespoon of oil over medium-high heat for 1 minute, or until shimmering.

4. Add the meatballs and sear, stirring occasionally to brown at least 2 sides, for 4 minutes. Transfer to a plate.

5. Add the remaining 1 teaspoon of oil to the pot.

6. Add the onion and garlic. Sauté, stirring occasionally, for 5 minutes, or until aromatic.

7. Add the broth, water, couscous, remaining ⅛ teaspoon of salt, and remaining ½ teaspoon of Italian seasoning. Bring to a boil.

8. Gently return the meatballs to the pot. Reduce the heat to medium. Cook for 10 minutes, or until the couscous is soft. Remove from the heat.

9. Add the spinach and cover the pot for 1 minute, or until the spinach has wilted.
10. Season the soup with the lemon juice and serve hot. Refrigerate leftovers in an airtight container for up to 4 days.

VARIATION TIP: Swap out the spinach for 1 cup chopped zucchini plus 1 cup chopped carrots. Because these veggies will take longer to cook than the spinach, be sure to add them during step 6 with the onion.

PER SERVING (¼ OF THE RECIPE): Calories: 479; Fat: 19g; Carbohydrates: 45g; Protein: 34g; Fiber: 3g; Sodium: 450mg; Iron: 3mg

BARBECUE TURKEY BOWLS

SERVES 4 | PREP TIME: 10 MINUTES **| COOK TIME:** 15 MINUTES

30-MINUTE MEAL | LEFTOVER-FRIENDLY | NUT-FREE

These zesty, flavorful bowls come together in a flash. Preparing your sweet potato in the microwave will save you significant cooking time, and tossing together a simple coleslaw keeps it a 30-minute meal. This way, you can focus on getting your turkey juicy and flavorful!

2 tablespoons olive oil, divided

12 ounces lean ground turkey

1 tablespoon DIY Taco Seasoning (page 198)

½ cup Date-Sweetened Barbecue Sauce (page 191)

½ cup plain low-fat Greek yogurt

Juice of 1 lemon

¼ teaspoon garlic powder

1 teaspoon honey

2 cups shredded cabbage

1 cup shredded carrots

¼ cup sliced Ginger Pickled Radish (page 200) (optional)

2 cups diced sweet potato

¼ cup water

4 butter lettuce leaves

1. In a large skillet, heat 1 tablespoon of oil over medium-high heat for 30 seconds, or until shimmering.

2. Add the ground turkey and taco seasoning. Cook, using a spatula to break the turkey into small pieces, for 7 to 9 minutes, or until browned throughout.

3. Mix in the barbecue sauce and cook for 1 to 2 minutes, or until warmed. Remove from the heat.

4. Meanwhile, prepare the coleslaw: In a large bowl, combine the yogurt, lemon juice, remaining 1 tablespoon of oil, the garlic powder, and honey.

5. Mix in the cabbage and carrots until well combined.

6. Garnish with the pickled radish (if using).

7. In a microwave-safe bowl, combine the sweet potato and water. Cover and microwave for 5 minutes, or until tender. Drain any excess water.

8. Place a lettuce leaf on one side of each of 4 bowls.

9. Fill each leaf with the turkey.

10. Add the sweet potato and coleslaw to the other side of the bowls. (The barbecue sauce adds a complementary flavor to all the components, so no need to worry if it gets on the coleslaw or sweet potato.) Refrigerate leftovers in separate airtight containers for up to 4 days.

VARIATION TIP: To give your coleslaw an extra kick, add 1 to 2 teaspoons DIY Taco Seasoning (page 198) to the blend. You can also use mayonnaise in the coleslaw instead of olive oil for more richness.

PER SERVING (¼ OF THE RECIPE): Calories: 468; Fat: 18g; Carbohydrates: 50g; Protein: 30g; Fiber: 8g; Sodium: 425mg; Iron: 4mg

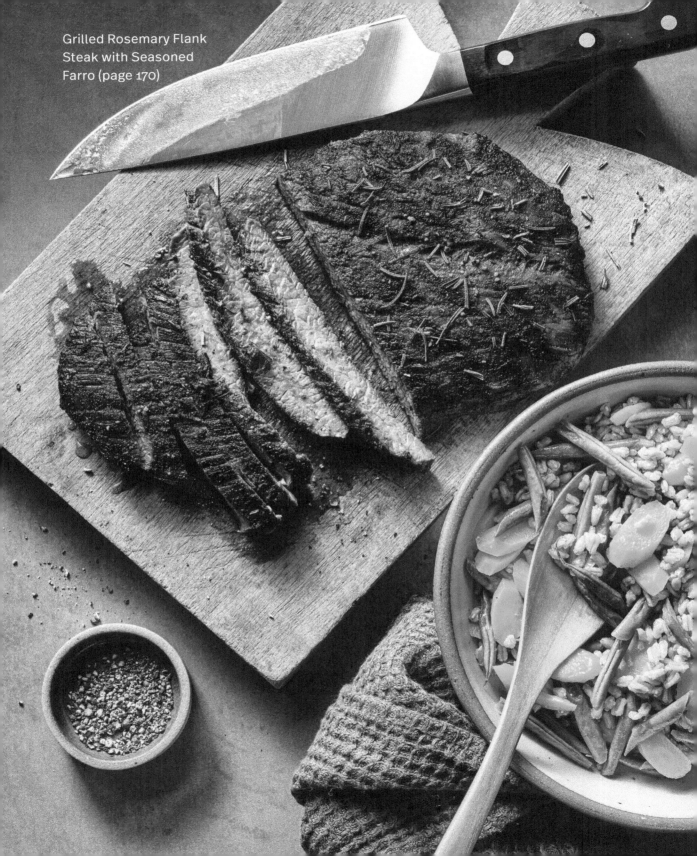

Grilled Rosemary Flank Steak with Seasoned Farro (page 170)

CHAPTER 8

PORK AND BEEF

Honey-Glazed Pork Chops **150**

Barbecue Pork Chops **152**

Pan-Seared Pork Chops with Kale, Corn, and Bell Pepper **154**

Spicy Chili Pork Bowls **156**

Teriyaki Pork Stir-Fry **157**

Pineapple Pork with Roasted Vegetables **158**

Stuffed Bell Peppers **160**

Barbecue-Glazed Meatloaf **162**

Beef and Mushroom Burgers **164**

Beef and Broccoli Stir-Fry **166**

Peppered Beef Macro Bowls **168**

Steak Salad with Sesame Dressing **169**

Grilled Rosemary Flank Steak with Seasoned Farro **170**

Lightened Beef Stroganoff **172**

HONEY-GLAZED PORK CHOPS

SERVES 4 | **PREP TIME:** 10 MINUTES | **COOK TIME:** 20 MINUTES

30-MINUTE MEAL | **LEFTOVER-FRIENDLY** | **NUT-FREE**

As these pork chops bake, they are bathed in the honey-balsamic glaze and their own natural juices. Basting halfway through the baking process keeps these chops flavorful, and searing before baking shortens the cooking time and adds a golden color.

2 tablespoons balsamic vinegar

¼ cup honey

4 (4-ounce) boneless pork chops

2½ tablespoons olive oil, divided

¼ teaspoon sea salt, divided

1⅓ cups dried couscous

2⅔ cups water

4 cups chopped lacinato kale

¼ teaspoon sea salt

PER SERVING (¼ OF THE RECIPE): Calories: 514; Fat: 13g; Carbohydrates: 64g; Protein: 34g; Fiber: 4g; Sodium: 227mg; Iron: 2mg

1. Place a large oven-safe skillet in the oven and preheat to 400°F. Line a 9-by-13-inch baking dish with aluminum foil.

2. In a small bowl, whisk together the vinegar and honey until well combined.

3. Put the pork chops, 1 tablespoon of oil, and ⅛ teaspoon of salt in a sealable plastic bag. Seal and shake vigorously to thoroughly coat.

4. Using oven mitts, carefully remove the hot skillet from the oven and set it on the stove; don't turn on the burner.

5. Pour ½ tablespoon of oil into the skillet and let it heat for 1 minute, then add the pork chops and sear them for 3 minutes per side or until golden brown.

6. Put the pork chops in the prepared baking dish, pour the glaze over top, and transfer to the oven. Bake for 8 to 10 minutes, basting the pork chops halfway through, until the internal temperature of the pork chops reaches 140°F. Remove from the oven.

7. Transfer the pork chops to a plate, pour any remaining juices over top, and cover loosely with foil. Let rest for at least 5 minutes, or until the internal temperature reaches 145°F.

8. Meanwhile, prepare the couscous. In a medium soup pot, combine the couscous and water. Bring to a boil over medium heat. Cook for 6 minutes, or until all the water has been absorbed. Remove from the heat.

9. While the couscous is cooking, in a medium skillet, heat the remaining 1 tablespoon of oil over medium heat for 1 minute, or until shimmering.

10. Add the kale and toss to coat. Cook, stirring occasionally, for 5 to 6 minutes, or until tender. Season with the remaining ⅛ teaspoon of salt. Remove from the heat.

11. Serve the pork over the kale with the couscous on the side. Pour any juices over top. Refrigerate leftovers separately in airtight containers for up to 4 days.

TECHNICAL TIP: Traditional small-grain couscous takes half the time of pearl couscous to cook, due to its tiny granular pieces.

BARBECUE PORK CHOPS

SERVES 4 | **PREP TIME:** 10 MINUTES | **COOK TIME:** 20 MINUTES

30-MINUTE MEAL | **LEFTOVER-FRIENDLY** | **NUT-FREE**

These pork chops are cooked on a rack over the carrots so the juices from the pork drip onto the carrots, adding a naturally flavorful glaze. With a head start in baking, the carrots should be done when the pork is ready.

4 (4-ounce) boneless pork chops

1 teaspoon, plus 1 tablespoon olive oil

¼ teaspoon sea salt

2 cups chopped carrots

1 cup Date-Sweetened Barbecue Sauce (page 191), divided

2 cups fresh or frozen green beans

¼ cup water

PER SERVING (¼ OF THE RECIPE): Calories: 310; Fat: 9g; Carbohydrates: 30g; Protein: 29g; Fiber: 7g; Sodium: 379mg; Iron: 2mg

1. Preheat the oven to 400°F. Line a 9-by-13-inch baking sheet with aluminum foil.

2. In a large, sealable plastic bag, combine the pork chops, 1 teaspoon of oil, and the salt. Seal and shake vigorously to thoroughly coat.

3. Spread the carrots out in a single layer on the prepared baking sheet.

4. Transfer the baking sheet to the oven and bake for about 10 minutes.

5. Meanwhile, in a large skillet, heat the remaining 1 tablespoon of oil over medium-high heat for 1 minute, or until shimmering.

6. Add the pork chops and sear for 3 minutes per side, or until golden brown. Remove from the heat.

7. Remove the baking sheet from the oven and set an oven-safe wire rack over the carrots. Place the pork on the rack.

8. Slather 3 tablespoons of barbecue sauce over each pork chop.

9. Return the baking sheet to the oven and bake the pork and carrots for 10 minutes, or until the internal temperature of the pork reaches 140°F. Remove from the oven. Transfer to a plate. Cover loosely with foil. Let rest for at least 5 minutes, or until the internal temperature reaches 145°F.

10. While the pork is baking, in a microwave-safe bowl, combine the green beans and water. Cover and microwave for 4 minutes, or until tender. Drain any excess water.

11. Serve the barbecue pork with the carrots and green beans. Serve the remaining ¼ cup of barbecue sauce for dipping. Refrigerate leftovers in an airtight container for up to 4 days.

TECHNICAL TIP: If you want to ensure juicy meat for this and other pork chop recipes, consider brining them prior to cooking. In a large bowl, dissolve 3 tablespoons sea salt in 1 cup boiling water. Add 2 cups cold water, then add the pork chops and soak for 30 minutes. Rinse and pat dry prior to preparation.

PAN-SEARED PORK CHOPS WITH KALE, CORN, AND BELL PEPPER

SERVES 4 | PREP TIME: 10 MINUTES | **COOK TIME:** 20 MINUTES

30-MINUTE MEAL | ONE POT/PAN | LEFTOVER-FRIENDLY | GLUTEN-FREE | NUT-FREE

When it comes to getting dinner on the table quickly, anything you can do to cut down on cook time makes a big difference. That's why this recipe uses the same skillet for both meat and veggies—you won't have to heat your skillet in the oven to speed up cook time, since it will already be hot from your sautéed veggies.

2 teaspoons olive oil, plus 1 tablespoon

2 cups frozen corn

2 cups frozen tricolor bell pepper strips

2 cups chopped lacinato kale

⅛ teaspoon sea salt, plus ¼ teaspoon

4 (4-ounce) boneless pork chops

1 teaspoon Italian or Tuscan seasoning

PER SERVING (¼ OF THE RECIPE): Calories: 294; Fat: 10g; Carbohydrates: 23g; Protein: 28g; Fiber: 6g; Sodium: 296mg; Iron: 2mg

1. In a large skillet, heat 2 teaspoons of oil over medium heat for 1 minute, or until shimmering.
2. Add the corn, bell pepper, and kale. Sauté for 5 to 6 minutes, or until all the veggies are tender and the kale is bright green. Transfer to a plate. Season with ⅛ teaspoon of salt.
3. Meanwhile, season the pork chops with the remaining ¼ teaspoon of salt and the Italian seasoning.
4. In the same skillet, heat the remaining 1 tablespoon of oil over medium-high heat for 1 minute, or until shimmering.

5. Add the pork chops and sear for 3 minutes per side, or until golden. Remove the skillet from the heat; leave the chops in the skillet to continue to cook for 2 minutes per side, or until the internal temperature reaches 140°F. Transfer to a cutting board. Let rest for at least 5 minutes, or until the pork's internal temperature reaches 145°F.

6. Thinly slice the pork chops, and serve with the vegetables. Refrigerate leftovers in an airtight container for up to 4 days.

TECHNICAL TIP: Letting the pork chops remain in the heated pan for a total of 4 minutes will ensure thorough cooking without scorching the surface. They'll finish cooking from the residual heat while they rest.

SPICY CHILI PORK BOWLS

SERVES 4 | PREP TIME: 15 MINUTES **| COOK TIME:** 10 MINUTES
30-MINUTE MEAL | LEFTOVER-FRIENDLY | GLUTEN-FREE

This dish kicks up some serious heat, so add a little more or less Sriracha sauce to your taste. Ginger pickled radish is a perfect garnish for this dish–for best results, you'll need to prepare it at least a day ahead to let the flavors mingle, so plan your meal accordingly.

5 tablespoons honey

2 tablespoons Sriracha sauce

2 teaspoons sesame oil or peanut oil

2 tablespoons apple cider vinegar

¼ cup low-fat mayonnaise

3 cups shredded cabbage

1 cup grated carrots

1 tablespoon olive oil

4 (4-ounce) boneless pork chops, cut into ½-inch dice

¼ teaspoon sea salt

2 cups frozen brown rice

½ cup chopped scallions, green parts only

20 slices Ginger Pickled Radish (page 200) (optional)

PER SERVING (¼ OF THE RECIPE): Calories: 405; Fat: 10g; Carbohydrates: 31g; Protein: 30g; Fiber: 4g; Sodium: 332mg; Iron: 1mg

1. In a small mixing bowl, whisk together the honey, Sriracha sauce, sesame oil, and vinegar.

2. In another bowl, toss ¼ cup of the Sriracha mixture with the mayonnaise, cabbage, and carrots.

3. In a large skillet, heat the olive oil over medium heat for 1 minute, or until shimmering.

4. Add the pork chops and cook, stirring occasionally, for 5 to 6 minutes, or until browned and cooked through. Season with the salt. Remove from the heat. Transfer to a medium bowl. Cover with aluminum foil to keep warm.

5. Prepare the rice in the microwave according to the package instructions, usually about 3 minutes.

6. Toss the remaining Sriracha mixture with the pork until evenly coated.

7. Divide the pork, cabbage mixture, and rice evenly among 4 bowls.

8. Garnish with the scallions and 5 pickled radish slices per bowl (if using). Refrigerate leftovers in an airtight container for 3 to 4 days.

INGREDIENT TIP: If you really love the heat, double up the Sriracha mixture, and refrigerate leftovers in an airtight container for up to 2 weeks.

TERIYAKI PORK STIR-FRY

SERVES 6 | PREP TIME: 10 MINUTES **| COOK TIME:** 15 MINUTES

30-MINUTE MEAL | LEFTOVER-FRIENDLY | NUT-FREE

This dish has that Japanese restaurant appeal while minimizing the added sugar and sodium. The date-sweetened teriyaki sauce delivers with its intense ginger-garlic-soy combo, and the high-heat cooking with small cuts of crunchy veggies keeps the cook time short.

3 tablespoons olive oil, divided

1½ cups thinly sliced carrots

3 cups small broccoli florets

3 cups frozen tricolor bell pepper strips

6 (4-ounce) boneless pork chops, cut into ½-inch dice

3 cups frozen brown rice

1½ cups Date-Sweetened Teriyaki Sauce (page 190)

PER SERVING (⅙ OF THE RECIPE): Calories: 412; Fat: 13g; Carbohydrates: 41g; Protein: 30g; Fiber: 8g; Sodium: 564mg; Iron: 3mg

1. In a large, high-sided skillet or wok, heat 2 tablespoons of oil over medium-high heat for 1 minute, or until shimmering.

2. Add the carrots, broccoli, and bell pepper. Cook, stirring occasionally, for 3 to 5 minutes, or until tender and slightly browned. Add 1 to 2 tablespoons of water as needed to keep the veggies from sticking. Transfer to a plate. Loosely cover with aluminum foil to keep warm.

3. In the same skillet, heat the remaining 1 tablespoon of oil for 1 minute, or until shimmering.

4. Add the pork chops and cook, stirring occasionally, for 5 to 6 minutes, or until browned and cooked through.

5. Meanwhile, prepare the rice in the microwave according to the package instructions, usually about 3 minutes. Divide among 6 bowls.

6. Return the veggies to the skillet. Add the teriyaki sauce and toss to fully coat. Remove from the heat.

7. Top each bowl with equal amounts of the pork and veggies. Refrigerate leftovers in an airtight container for up to 4 days.

PINEAPPLE PORK WITH ROASTED VEGETABLES

SERVES 4 | **PREP TIME:** 10 MINUTES | **COOK TIME:** 20 MINUTES

30-MINUTE MEAL | **ONE POT/PAN** | **LEFTOVER-FRIENDLY**

A one-pot meal, this pineapple pork will keep cleanup convenient and your cook time relatively short. You'll simply bake everything on the same tray all at once, allowing the juices from the pork, pineapple, and sesame dressing to season the vegetables.

4 (4-ounce) boneless pork chops

¼ cup Sesame Dressing (page 193)

½ teaspoon sea salt, divided

2 medium russet potatoes, quartered and cut widthwise into ⅛-inch pieces

2 cups small broccoli florets, coarsely chopped

2 cups chopped carrots

¼ teaspoon dried rosemary

½ teaspoon garlic powder

1 tablespoon olive oil

4 canned pineapple rings

PER SERVING (¼ OF THE RECIPE): Calories: 350; Fat: 9g; Carbohydrates: 36g; Protein: 30g; Fiber: 5g; Sodium: 533mg; Iron: 2mg

1. Preheat the oven to 425°F. Line a 9-by-13-inch baking sheet with aluminum foil.

2. In a large, sealable plastic bag, combine the pork chops, dressing, and ¼ teaspoon of salt. Seal and shake well to coat.

3. Spread the potatoes, broccoli, and carrots out on the prepared baking sheet in a single layer, making space in the center for the chops.

4. Sprinkle the veggies with the remaining ¼ teaspoon of salt, the rosemary, and garlic powder. Drizzle the oil on top.

5. Place the pork chops in the center of the baking sheet.

6. Place a pineapple ring on top of each.

7. Transfer the baking sheet to the oven and bake for 20 minutes, or until the internal temperature of the pork reaches 140°F and the vegetables are tender. Remove from the oven. (You can leave the vegetables in the oven to cook a little longer if you prefer them very tender.) Transfer the pork to a plate. Cover loosely with foil for 5 minutes, or until the internal temperature reaches 145°F. Refrigerate leftovers in an airtight container for 4 days.

VARIATION TIP: For an alternative glaze for the pork, whisk ¼ cup honey with 2 tablespoons soy sauce and use it in place of the sesame dressing.

STUFFED BELL PEPPERS

SERVES 6 | PREP TIME: 10 MINUTES **| COOK TIME:** 20 MINUTES

30-MINUTE MEAL | LEFTOVER-FRIENDLY | NUT-FREE

Seasoned meat and rice in a bell pepper pocket is always fun! Top it with some parmesan, and it's even better—definitely a choice that kids will love. The bell peppers are par-cooked in the microwave to save overall time.

6 medium bell peppers, tops removed, cored

⅓ cup water

1 tablespoon olive oil

12 ounces (80 percent lean) ground beef

⅛ teaspoon sea salt

1 teaspoon garlic powder

1 teaspoon Italian seasoning

1½ cups low-sodium marinara sauce

6 cups baby spinach

3 cups frozen brown rice

¾ cup grated parmesan cheese

PER SERVING (⅙ OF THE RECIPE): Calories: 353; Fat: 16g; Carbohydrates: 31g; Protein: 23g; Fiber: 6g; Sodium: 411mg; Iron: 4mg

1. Preheat the oven to 450°F. Line a 9-by-13-inch baking sheet with aluminum foil.

2. Place the bell peppers, face up, in a large, microwave-safe bowl with the water. Cover and microwave for 5 minutes, or until tender. Drain.

3. Meanwhile, place a large, oven-safe skillet inside the oven for 2 minutes. Using oven mitts, transfer to the stove.

4. In the skillet, heat the oil over medium-high heat for 1 minute, or until shimmering.

5. Add the ground beef and use a spatula to break it into small pieces. Season with the salt, garlic powder, and Italian seasoning. Cook for 5 to 7 minutes, or until thoroughly browned.

6. Add the marinara and spinach. Cover the skillet and cook for 2 minutes, or until the spinach has wilted. Remove from the heat.

7. Meanwhile, prepare the rice in the microwave according to the package instructions, usually about 3 minutes.

8. Assemble the bell peppers on the prepared baking sheet: evenly fill each pepper with the rice and ground beef mixture.

9. Top each with 2 tablespoons of cheese.

10. Transfer the baking sheet to the oven and bake for 5 minutes, or until the cheese has melted. Remove from the oven. Refrigerate leftovers in an airtight container for up to 4 days.

VARIATION TIP: For an alternative to rice, try pearl couscous. You can prepare it on the stove separately while the meat cooks.

BARBECUE-GLAZED MEATLOAF

SERVES 4 | **PREP TIME:** 15 MINUTES | **COOK TIME:** 1 HOUR 10 MINUTES

LEFTOVER-FRIENDLY | **NUT-FREE**

Meatloaf—it's one of those traditional comfort foods, and a perfect addition to your family meal repertoire. Date-sweetened barbecue sauce replaces the standard ketchup topping for a zesty tang, and a bit of Worcestershire adds to the umami flavor.

Nonstick cooking spray, for coating

1½ tablespoons olive oil, divided

½ cup 5-Ingredient Mirepoix (page 199)

1 pound (80 percent lean) ground beef

½ cup panko bread crumbs

1 medium egg

1 tablespoon low-sodium Worcestershire sauce

1 teaspoon garlic powder

¼ teaspoon sea salt, plus ⅛ teaspoon

2 tablespoons Date-Sweetened Barbecue Sauce (page 191), plus ½ cup

12 baby potatoes

2 cups fresh or frozen green beans

¼ cup water

2 tablespoons chopped fresh parsley (optional)

1. Preheat the oven to 350°F. Line a 5-by-9-inch loaf pan with parchment paper or aluminum foil. Coat lightly with cooking spray.

2. In a medium skillet, heat ½ tablespoon of olive oil over medium heat for 1 minute, or until shimmering.

3. Add the mirepoix and sauté for 5 to 7 minutes, or until softened. Remove from the heat.

4. In a large bowl, combine the beef, bread crumbs, egg, Worcestershire sauce, garlic powder, ¼ teaspoon of salt, mirepoix, and 2 tablespoons of barbecue sauce. Using your hands, mash until well combined. Transfer to the prepared loaf pan. Mold with a slightly domed top.

5. Slather with the remaining ½ cup of barbecue sauce.

6. Transfer the loaf pan to the oven and bake for 1 hour, or until the internal temperature reaches 160°F. Remove from the oven. Let rest for 10 minutes before slicing.

7. Meanwhile, in a medium soup pot, combine the potatoes with enough water to fully cover. Bring to a boil over medium-high heat.

8. Reduce the heat to medium. Cook for 10 to 15 minutes, or until the potatoes are tender. Remove from the heat. Transfer to a cutting board. Slice in half lengthwise. In a large, sealable plastic bag or medium bowl, toss with the remaining 1 tablespoon of olive oil and ⅛ teaspoon of salt.

9. In a microwave-safe bowl, combine the green beans and water. Cover and microwave for 4 minutes, or until tender. Drain any excess water.

10. Serve the meatloaf with the potatoes and green beans.

11. Garnish with the parsley (if using). Refrigerate leftovers in an airtight container for up to 4 days.

SUBSTITUTION TIP: You can swap out the panko for an equal amount of instant mashed potato flakes if you like.

PER SERVING (¼ OF THE RECIPE): Calories: 417; Fat: 17g; Carbohydrates: 44g; Protein: 25g; Fiber: 5g; Sodium: 379mg; Iron: 4mg

BEEF AND MUSHROOM BURGERS

SERVES 4 | **PREP TIME:** 10 MINUTES | **COOK TIME:** 25 MINUTES

NUT-FREE

You get a few more veggies in this meal with the addition of sautéed mushrooms blended into your beef patties. Served with lemon-caper aïoli on whole-wheat buns, these burgers have got all the fixings for a mouthwatering meal.

4 teaspoons plus 1 tablespoon olive oil, divided

4 cups chopped lacinato kale

¼ teaspoon sea salt, divided

2½ cups finely chopped white mushrooms

¼ cup chopped scallions, both white and green parts

1 pound (80 percent lean) ground beef

1½ tablespoons low-sodium Worcestershire sauce

1 teaspoon garlic powder

4 medium whole-wheat hamburger buns

8 tablespoons Lemon-Caper Aïoli (page 197)

1. In a large skillet, heat 2 teaspoons of oil over medium-high heat for 1 minute, or until shimmering.

2. Add the kale, toss until well coated, and sauté for 3 minutes, or until tender and lightly crisp on the edges. Transfer to a plate. Season with ⅛ teaspoon of salt.

3. Reduce the heat to medium. Heat 2 teaspoons of oil for 30 seconds, or until shimmering.

4. Add the mushrooms and sauté for 5 to 7 minutes, or until tender and reduced in size by half.

5. Stir in the scallions and cook for 1 minute, or until fragrant. Remove from the heat. Transfer to a large bowl.

6. Add the beef, Worcestershire sauce, garlic powder, and remaining ⅛ teaspoon of salt. Mash well to combine.

7. Form the mixture into 4 equal patties.

8. In the same skillet, heat the remaining 1 tablespoon of oil over medium-high heat for 30 seconds, or until shimmering.

9. Add the patties and cook for 3 to 5 minutes per side, or until they reach your desired doneness. Transfer to a plate. Cover loosely with aluminum foil to keep warm.

10. Add the buns to the skillet and toast for about 1 minute. Remove from the heat.

11. Spread 2 tablespoons of aïoli onto each bun and sandwich the patties. Serve with the sautéed kale.

VARIATION TIP: For a zesty alternative, swap out the Lemon-Caper Aïoli for Date-Sweetened Barbecue Sauce (page 191), or keep it simple with just ketchup.

PER SERVING (¼ OF THE RECIPE): Calories: 523; Fat: 25g; Carbohydrates: 37g; Protein: 38g; Fiber: 6g; Sodium: 614mg; Iron: 6mg

BEEF AND BROCCOLI STIR-FRY

SERVES 6 | PREP TIME: 10 MINUTES **| COOK TIME:** 15 MINUTES

30-MINUTE MEAL | LEFTOVER-FRIENDLY | NUT-FREE

Enjoy one of your favorite Chinese restaurant dishes at home. Cornstarch not only thickens the sauce but also gives your whole dish that glossy look. Par-cooking the broccoli in the microwave will keep it bright green and shorten the overall cook time.

5 tablespoons
   cornstarch, divided

6 tablespoons water,
   plus ¼ cup

1½ pounds flank
   steak, cubed

6 tablespoons low-sodium
   soy sauce

3 tablespoons honey

1 tablespoon minced garlic

1 tablespoon finely grated
   fresh ginger root

3 tablespoons olive
   oil, divided

6 cups small
   broccoli florets

3 cups frozen brown rice

PER SERVING (⅙ OF THE RECIPE): Calories: 405; Fat: 15g; Carbohydrates: 37g; Protein: 30g; Fiber: 3g; Sodium: 689mg; Iron: 3mg

1. In a large bowl, whisk together 4 tablespoons of cornstarch and 6 tablespoons of water until a thin paste forms.

2. Add the steak and toss to coat well.

3. To make the sauce, in a small bowl, whisk together the soy sauce, honey, garlic, ginger, and remaining 1 tablespoon of cornstarch until well combined.

4. In a large skillet or wok, heat 1½ tablespoons of oil over medium-high heat for 1 minute, or until shimmering.

5. Add the steak and cook, stirring occasionally, for about 5 minutes, or until nearly cooked through. Remove from the heat. Transfer to a plate. Cover loosely with aluminum foil to keep warm.

6. Meanwhile, in a microwave-safe bowl, combine the broccoli and remaining ¼ cup of water. Cover and microwave for 3 minutes, or until beginning to soften. Drain.

7. Prepare the rice in the microwave according to the package instructions, usually about 3 minutes.

8. In the same skillet, heat the remaining 1½ tablespoons of oil for 30 seconds, or until shimmering.

9. Add the broccoli and stir-fry for 5 minutes, or until tender.

10. Return the steak to the skillet. Add the sauce and cook for 1 minute, or until it starts to bubble and thicken. Remove from the heat.

11. Serve the broccoli beef over the rice. Refrigerate leftovers in an airtight container for up to 4 days.

VARIATION TIP: For an alternative to rice, serve the broccoli and beef with a side of corn.

PEPPERED BEEF MACRO BOWLS

SERVES 4 | **PREP TIME:** 15 MINUTES | **COOK TIME:** 20 MINUTES
ONE POT/PAN | **LEFTOVER-FRIENDLY** | **GLUTEN-FREE** | **NUT-FREE**

Seasoned beef, sautéed Brussels sprouts, and sweet potato medallions make this bowl complete with a good distribution of macronutrients. Creamy cilantro dressing drizzled on top brings it all together with flavorful tang and brightness.

2 tablespoons olive oil, divided

1 pound lean flank steak, cut against the grain into small strips

1 teaspoon lemon pepper seasoning

¼ teaspoon sea salt

4 cups small Brussels sprouts, trimmed and halved

1 recipe Sweet Potato Medallions (page 203)

½ cup Creamy Cilantro Dressing (page 194)

PER SERVING (¼ OF THE RECIPE): Calories: 428; Fat: 21g; Carbohydrates: 30g; Protein: 32g; Fiber: 7g; Sodium: 552mg; Iron: 4mg

1. In a large skillet, heat 1 tablespoon of oil over medium-high heat for 1 minute, or until shimmering.

2. Add the steak and stir-fry for about 5 minutes for medium-well, or to your desired doneness (keeping in mind it will continue to cook as it rests). Transfer to a plate. Season with the lemon pepper. Cover loosely with aluminum foil to keep warm.

3. To the skillet, add the remaining 1 tablespoon of oil, the salt, and the Brussels sprouts.

4. Reduce the heat to medium-low. Cook for 8 minutes, undisturbed. Then continue to cook, stirring occasionally, for another 5 minutes, or until the Brussels sprouts are browned and tender. Remove from the heat.

5. Layer the beef, Brussels sprouts, and sweet potato medallions in 4 bowls.

6. Drizzle the dressing on top and serve. Refrigerate leftovers in an airtight container for up to 3 days.

VARIATION TIP: Swap out the Brussels sprouts for chopped asparagus. You'll prepare them the same way.

STEAK SALAD WITH SESAME DRESSING

SERVES 4 | **PREP TIME:** 15 MINUTES | **COOK TIME:** 10 MINUTES
30-MINUTE MEAL | **LEFTOVER-FRIENDLY**

This salad is delicious with sesame dressing, but it's easily inter-changeable—any vinaigrette will do. Try my Lemon-Basil Vinaigrette (page 192) for another flavorful option.

2 tablespoons cornstarch

3 tablespoons water, plus ¼ cup

1 pound lean flank steak, cut against the grain into small strips

1 tablespoon olive oil

⅛ teaspoon sea salt

1 cup frozen corn

4 cups chopped romaine lettuce

4 small vine-ripened tomatoes, cut into quarters

¼ cup chopped scallions, green parts only

2 to 3 tablespoons Sesame Dressing (page 193)

2 tablespoons sesame seeds (optional)

PER SERVING (¼ OF THE RECIPE): Calories: 339; Fat: 14g; Carbohydrates: 26g; Protein: 29g; Fiber: 5g; Sodium: 369mg; Iron: 3mg

1. In a large bowl, whisk together the cornstarch and 3 tablespoons of water into a thin paste.
2. Add the steak and toss to coat well.
3. In a large skillet or wok, heat the oil over medium-high heat for 1 minute, or until shimmering.
4. Add the steak in 1 layer and stir-fry for about 5 minutes for medium-well, or to your desired doneness. Remove from the heat. Transfer to a plate. Season with the salt. Cover loosely with aluminum foil to keep warm.
5. In a microwave-safe bowl, combine the corn and remaining ¼ cup of water. Cover and micro-wave for 3 minutes. Drain any excess water.
6. In a large salad bowl, toss together the lettuce, corn, tomatoes, scallions, and dressing. Divide among 4 bowls.
7. Top with equal portions of the steak.
8. Garnish with the sesame seeds (if using). Refrig-erate leftover steak in an airtight container for 3 to 4 days.

TECHNICAL TIP: The steak will continue to cook while resting, so if you prefer it medium-well rather than well done, shorten your cook time by a minute or two.

GRILLED ROSEMARY FLANK STEAK WITH SEASONED FARRO

SERVES 4 | **PREP TIME:** 10 MINUTES, PLUS 30 MINUTES TO MARINATE |
COOK TIME: 30 TO 35 MINUTES

LEFTOVER-FRIENDLY | **NUT-FREE**

This steak is marinated with rosemary and garlic to mirror the flavors of the seasoned farro, then grilled to perfection in just minutes.

Nonstick cooking spray, for coating the grill

¼ cup olive oil

2 tablespoons low-sodium Worcestershire sauce

Juice of ½ lemon

2 teaspoons honey

¼ teaspoon dried rosemary, divided

½ teaspoon garlic powder, divided

1 pound lean flank steak

1 cup farro

1½ cups low-sodium chicken or beef broth

1¼ cups water, divided

⅛ teaspoon sea salt

1 cup fresh or frozen trimmed green beans

1 cup sliced carrots

2 tablespoons plain low-fat Greek yogurt, for garnish (optional)

1. Preheat an outdoor grill to medium-high heat. Lightly coat with cooking spray.

2. In a large, sealable plastic bag, combine the oil, Worcestershire sauce, lemon juice, honey, ⅛ teaspoon of rosemary, and ¼ teaspoon of garlic powder.

3. Add the steak, seal, and massage to fully coat. Refrigerate for 30 minutes to marinate.

4. Meanwhile, in a medium soup pot, combine the farro, broth, and 1 cup of water. Bring to a boil over medium-high heat.

5. Reduce the heat to medium-low. Cover the pot and simmer for 15 to 20 minutes, or until the farro is tender yet chewy. Remove from the heat. Drain any excess liquid. Season with the remaining ⅛ teaspoon of rosemary, ¼ teaspoon of garlic powder, and the salt. Lightly fluff with a fork.

6. Put the steak on the grill and cook for 6 minutes per side for medium-well, or to your desired doneness. Remove from the heat. Let rest for 5 to 10 minutes.

7. While the steak is resting, in a microwave-safe dish, combine the green beans, carrots, and remaining ¼ cup of water. Cover and microwave for 4 minutes, or until tender. Drain any excess water.

8. Cut the steak against the grain into ¼-inch-thick slices.

9. Top with a dollop of yogurt per serving (if using).

10. Serve the steak with the farro and veggies. Refrigerate leftovers in an airtight container for up to 4 days.

VARIATION TIP: For a veggie variation, in a microwave-safe dish, combine 4 cups halved Brussels sprouts and ¼ cup water. Cover and microwave for 4 minutes. Then place the Brussels sprouts on the preheated grill and cook for 3 to 5 minutes, or until browned on the edges.

PER SERVING (¼ OF THE RECIPE): Calories: 550; Fat: 22g; Carbohydrates: 57g; Protein: 35g; Fiber: 10g; Sodium: 174mg; Iron: 5mg

LIGHTENED BEEF STROGANOFF

SERVES 4 | **PREP TIME:** 10 MINUTES | **COOK TIME:** 20 MINUTES

30-MINUTE MEAL | **LEFTOVER-FRIENDLY** | **NUT-FREE**

With cream of mushroom soup instead of heavy cream and butter, this is a lighter version of the comforting classic. It's also a veggie-rich version with sautéed bell pepper, mushrooms, onions, and spinach.

2 tablespoons olive oil

1½ cups chopped yellow onions

1 cup chopped white mushrooms

1 cup chopped red bell pepper

2 teaspoons minced garlic

8 ounces lean flank steak, cut against the grain into thin strips

1 (10½-ounce) can low-sodium cream of mushroom soup

1 cup low-sodium beef broth

2 teaspoons low-sodium Worcestershire sauce

2 cups baby spinach

⅛ teaspoon sea salt

Freshly ground black pepper

8 ounces dried egg noodles

¼ cup chopped fresh parsley

1. In a large skillet, heat the oil over medium-high heat for 1 minute, or until shimmering.
2. Add the onions, mushrooms, bell pepper, and garlic.
3. Reduce the heat to medium. Cook, stirring occasionally, for 5 to 7 minutes, or until the onions and bell pepper are tender. Transfer to a plate.
4. Increase the heat to medium. Add the steak to the skillet. Cook for 5 to 6 minutes, or until browned.
5. Stir in the cream of mushroom soup, broth, and Worcestershire sauce.
6. Return the onions and bell pepper to the skillet. Bring to a boil.
7. Add the spinach. Remove from the heat. Cover the skillet until the spinach has wilted. Season with the salt and pepper.

8. Meanwhile, in a medium soup pot, bring plenty of water to a boil over medium-high heat.

9. Add the noodles to the pot and cook for 10 to 12 minutes, or until tender. Remove from the heat. Drain.

10. Divide the cooked noodles among 4 bowls, then pour the beef stroganoff over top. Garnish with the parsley. Refrigerate leftovers in an airtight container for up to 4 days.

VARIATION TIP: To make it more like a stew, swap out the egg noodles for 1 cup dried farro (cover the pot and cook for 15 to 20 minutes in step 9 if using this option).

PER SERVING (¼ OF THE RECIPE): Calories: 394; Fat: 9g; Carbohydrates: 55g; Protein: 24g; Fiber: 4g; Sodium: 195mg; Iron: 5mg

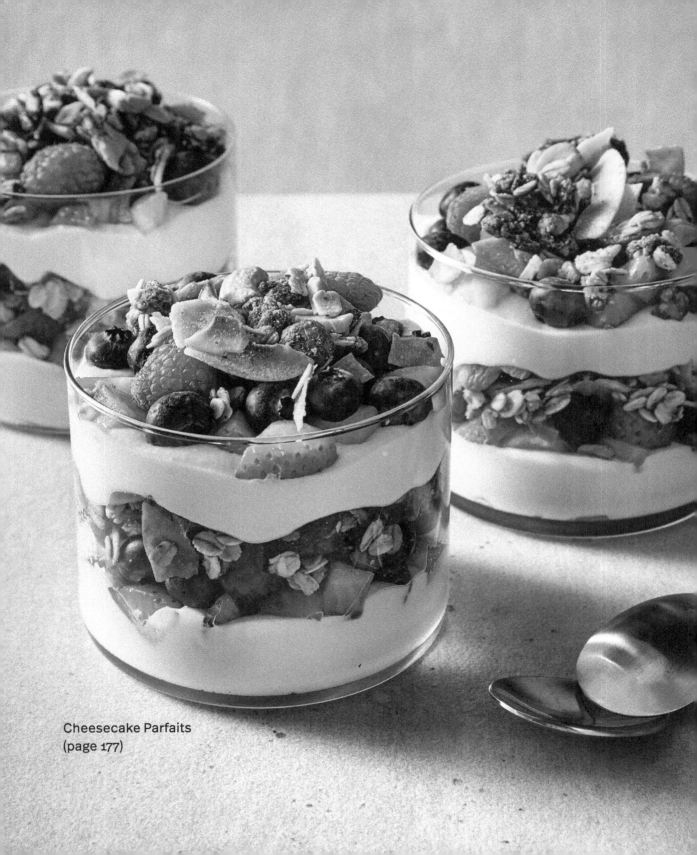

Cheesecake Parfaits
(page 177)

CHAPTER 9

DESSERTS

Lemon-Blueberry
Parfaits **176**

Cheesecake Parfaits **177**

Chocolate-Avocado
Pudding **178**

Strawberries and
Cream **179**

Honey-Almond Energy
Bites **180**

Peanut Butter and
Chocolate Chip
Cookies **181**

Coconut-Almond
Macaroons **182**

Lemon-Ricotta
Cupcakes **184**

Maple-Tahini Brownies **185**

Maple-Sesame Oat Cake
with Blueberry Topping **186**

LEMON–BLUEBERRY PARFAITS

SERVES 4 | **PREP TIME:** 20 MINUTES, PLUS 30 MINUTES TO CHILL | **COOK TIME:** 5 MINUTES

NUT-FREE | **VEGETARIAN**

This dessert features the fresh essence of lemon zest and wild blueberries, which have a more intense flavor than traditional blueberries. They are also packed with 33 percent more antho-cyanins–pigment-rich antioxidants that support brain health. The turmeric adds to the rich yellow color, but if you'd like to activate some of its anti-inflammatory curcumin, add a pinch of black pepper.

¼ cup freshly squeezed lemon juice (about 2 lemons)

3 tablespoons honey

½ cup unsweetened oat milk or soy milk

⅛ teaspoon turmeric

1 tablespoon cornstarch

1 to 2 teaspoons grated lemon zest

⅛ teaspoon sea salt

⅛ teaspoon freshly ground black pepper (optional)

1 cup plain low-fat Greek yogurt

1 cup frozen wild blueberries, slightly thawed

PER SERVING (ABOUT ½ CUP): Calories: 142; Fat: 2g; Carbohydrates: 26g; Protein: 7g; Fiber: 2g; Sodium: 110mg; Iron: 1mg

1. To make the curd, in a small pot, combine the lemon juice, honey, oat milk, and turmeric. Whisk briskly over medium heat for about 1 minute, or until thoroughly combined.

2. Add the cornstarch and whisk for 3 to 4 minutes, or until the curd thickens. Remove from the heat. Transfer to a bowl. Let sit at room temperature for about 15 minutes, or until cool. Then cover and refrigerate for 30 minutes until well chilled.

3. Stir in the lemon zest, salt, and pepper (if using).

4. Assemble 4 jars with alternating layers of lemon curd, yogurt, and wild blueberries.

CHEESECAKE PARFAITS

SERVES 4 | PREP TIME: 15 MINUTES, PLUS 30 MINUTES TO CHILL

VEGETARIAN

This creamy parfait has all the flavor of cheesecake but takes a fraction of the time to prepare. Assembled with mixed berries and maple-date granola, this cheesecake parfait is a simple, delightful combo kids and adults will all enjoy.

¾ cup plain low-fat Greek yogurt

¾ cup part-skim ricotta cheese

¼ cup low-fat whipped cream cheese

1 tablespoon honey

1 cup mixed frozen berries, slightly thawed

½ recipe Maple-Date Granola (page 40)

½ teaspoon ground cinnamon

PER SERVING (1 PARFAIT):
Calories: 256; Fat: 10g; Carbohydrates: 31g; Protein: 13g; Fiber: 3g; Sodium: 136mg; Iron: 1mg

1. To make the cheesecake mixture, in a medium bowl, whisk together the yogurt, ricotta cheese, cream cheese, and honey until creamy.

2. Assemble 4 jars with alternating layers of the cheesecake mixture, berries, and granola. Chill for 30 minutes in the refrigerator.

3. Dust with the cinnamon before serving.

VARIATION TIP: To save some time, you can use a low-sugar granola instead of making your own. Just be sure it has no more than 6 grams of added sugars per serving. Some good options include 18 Rabbits, Bear Naked, and Purely Elizabeth brands.

CHOCOLATE-AVOCADO PUDDING

SERVES 4 | PREP TIME: 5 MINUTES

30-MINUTE MEAL | ONE POT/PAN | GLUTEN-FREE | NUT-FREE | VEGAN

This creamy chocolate pudding has the benefit of fiber-rich avocado (a medium avocado contains about 10 grams of fiber). In addition to its high fiber content and monounsaturated (healthy) fats, avocado is also a good source of glutathione, an antioxidant that is necessary for the body's natural detoxification process.

2 medium ripe avocados, pitted and peeled

¼ cup unsweetened cocoa powder

¼ teaspoon ground cinnamon

6 tablespoons unsweetened soy milk

¼ teaspoon vanilla extract

¼ teaspoon sea salt

4 small, pitted dates

PER SERVING (ABOUT ½ CUP): Calories: 154; Fat: 12g; Carbohydrates: 15g; Protein: 3g; Fiber: 8g; Sodium: 161mg; Iron: 1mg

In a blender, combine the avocados, cocoa powder, cinnamon, soy milk, vanilla, salt, and dates. Process until well combined. Serve immediately.

VARIATION TIP: To make this even more chocolatey, add ½ teaspoon finely ground coffee to the mix. Coffee brings out the intensity of the chocolate.

STRAWBERRIES AND CREAM

SERVES 4 | PREP TIME: 5 MINUTES, PLUS 8 HOURS TO SOAK

LEFTOVER-FRIENDLY | GLUTEN-FREE | VEGAN

Strawberries and cream are a classic combo. This version uses a homemade vegan cream made with soaked cashews. The nuts are mild, making them perfect for creating a creamy base. Nutritionally, they are a good source of iron, zinc, and healthy fats. Be sure to soak your cashews overnight for the best possible texture.

½ cup whole raw cashews

¾ cup water, divided

2 small pitted dates

1/16 teaspoon sea salt

3 cups halved strawberries

¼ teaspoon ground cinnamon (optional)

PER SERVING (¾ CUP STRAWBERRIES + 2 TABLESPOONS CASHEW CREAM): Calories: 137; Fat: 8g; Carbohydrates: 17g; Protein: 4g; Fiber: 3g; Sodium: 43mg; Iron: 2mg

1. Put the cashews and ½ cup of water in an airtight jar. Refrigerate for 8 hours or overnight, then drain and rinse.

2. To make the cashew cream, in a blender, combine the soaked cashews, remaining ¼ cup of water, the dates, and salt. Process until creamy and smooth.

3. Divide the strawberries among 4 serving bowls.

4. Top with 2 tablespoons of cashew cream.

5. Dust with the cinnamon (if using).

SUBSTITUTION TIP: Don't have strawberries? This treat works with most berries. Try raspberries, blueberries, blackberries, or a combination.

TECHNICAL TIP: If you don't have time to soak the cashews overnight, you can simply put them in a microwave-safe bowl with an equal amount of water, then cover and microwave for 4 minutes to soften them same day. They'll soak up enough water to blend, but they won't be quite as smooth as if you'd soaked them overnight.

HONEY–ALMOND ENERGY BITES

MAKES 16 ENERGY BITES | **PREP TIME:** 10 MINUTES, PLUS 30 MINUTES TO CHILL

LEFTOVER-FRIENDLY | **VEGETARIAN**

These tasty energy bites are so easy to make, and there is no baking involved. Simply mix, form into balls, and enjoy! For best results, chill the batter before you roll it into balls–it's less sticky and easier to form the bites this way.

½ cup sliced almonds

½ cup almond butter or all-natural peanut butter

⅓ cup honey

1 cup rolled oats

¼ cup unsweetened coconut flakes

PER SERVING (2 ENERGY BITES): Calories: 217; Fat: 11g; Carbohydrates: 28g; Protein: 5g; Fiber: 3g; Sodium: 37mg; Iron: 1mg

1. Put the almonds in a small sealable plastic bag. Seal, and using a rolling pin, crush well.

2. In a medium bowl, combine the crushed almonds, almond butter, honey, oats, and coconut flakes until well incorporated. Cover and chill in the refrigerator for 30 minutes.

3. Roll the mixture into bite-size balls. Enjoy immediately, or refrigerate in an airtight container for up to 1 week.

VARIATION TIP: Swap out the coconut for an equal portion of almond meal to give these bites even more almond-y delight.

PEANUT BUTTER AND CHOCOLATE CHIP COOKIES

MAKES 18 COOKIES | **PREP TIME:** 10 MINUTES | **COOK TIME:** 10 MINUTES
30-MINUTE MEAL | **LEFTOVER-FRIENDLY** | **VEGETARIAN**

Date-sweetened with just a bit of honey, these cookies are packed with whole-food ingredients—including almonds and naturally sweet coconut.

Nonstick cooking spray, for coating the baking sheet

½ cup all-natural peanut butter

16 small, pitted dates

3 tablespoons canola oil

1 tablespoon honey

1 medium egg

1 cup rolled oats

½ cup raw, unsalted almonds or almond meal

½ cup unsweetened shredded coconut

¼ cup all-purpose flour

1 teaspoon baking soda

½ teaspoon sea salt

½ cup chocolate chips

PER SERVING (1 COOKIE):
Calories: 171; Fat: 11g; Carbohydrates: 16g; Protein: 4g; Fiber: 2g; Sodium: 162mg; Iron: 1mg

1. Preheat the oven to 375°F. Coat a baking sheet with cooking spray.
2. To make the batter, in a food processor, combine the peanut butter, dates, canola oil, honey, and egg. Process until smooth and creamy.
3. Add the oats, almonds, shredded coconut, flour, baking soda, and salt. Continue to process until well combined. (It's okay if there are some date flecks.) Transfer the batter to a bowl.
4. Mix in the chocolate chips.
5. Using a rounded tablespoon or a mini (1-ounce) ice cream scoop, scoop the batter, 2 inches apart, onto the prepared baking sheet.
6. Transfer the baking sheet to the oven and bake for 8 to 10 minutes, or until the edges are firm and golden and the bottoms have lightly browned. Remove from the oven. Place on a wire rack to cool for 5 to 10 minutes before serving. Store leftovers in an airtight container at room temperature for up to 3 days.

VARIATION TIP: To make these cookies nut-free, use sunflower seed butter, omit the almonds, and double up on the coconut.

COCONUT-ALMOND MACAROONS

MAKES 16 MACAROONS | PREP TIME: 10 MINUTES **| COOK TIME:** 15 MINUTES
30-MINUTE MEAL | GLUTEN-FREE | VEGETARIAN

If you are looking to cut refined sugars, these macaroons are a whole food–inspired treat that relies on dates and a bit of maple syrup incorporated at the end to achieve an ideal balance of flavor and sweetness.

1 cup unsweetened coconut flakes

¾ cup almond meal

8 small, pitted dates

½ teaspoon ground cinnamon

¼ teaspoon sea salt

4 medium egg whites

2 tablespoons maple syrup

**PER SERVING
(2 MACAROONS):** Calories: 141; Fat: 9g; Carbohydrates: 12g; Protein: 4g; Fiber: 3g; Sodium: 86mg; Iron: 1mg

1. Preheat the oven to 350°F. Line a baking sheet with parchment paper.

2. Put the coconut flakes, almond meal, dates, cinnamon, and salt in a food processor. Process until well combined. It's okay to have small flecks of dates peeking through the mixture. Transfer to a medium bowl.

3. In a separate medium bowl, using a handheld electric mixer, whip the egg whites on high speed until they form soft peaks. To make the dough, gently fold into the coconut-almond mixture until most of the fluff disappears into the mixture.

4. Slowly drizzle in the maple syrup as you mix.

5. Using a mini (1-ounce) ice cream scoop or a soup spoon, scoop the dough into mounds 2 inches apart on the prepared baking sheet. Pinch the tops to make peaks.

6. Transfer the baking sheet to the oven and bake for 12 to 15 minutes, or until the macaroons are firm and lightly browned on the edges. Remove from the oven. Transfer to a wire rack to cool for 5 to 10 minutes before serving. (If the peaks have fallen during baking, simply pinch after you take the macaroons out of the oven, and they will hold their shape as they cool.)

TECHNICAL TIP: Although you may be tempted to process all the ingredients together, whipping the egg whites before folding into the mixture adds lightness, and slowly adding the maple syrup at the end allows the egg white mixture to fully incorporate without forming lumps in the batter.

LEMON-RICOTTA CUPCAKES

MAKES 12 CUPCAKES | PREP TIME: 10 MINUTES | **COOK TIME:** 20 MINUTES

30-MINUTE MEAL | LEFTOVER-FRIENDLY | NUT-FREE | VEGETARIAN

Lemon and ricotta is such a delightful combo in this portion-friendly and kid-friendly treat. Be sure to zest your lemon before you juice it. The zest will be used in the batter and in the frosting.

Nonstick cooking spray, for coating

1½ cups part-skim ricotta cheese

⅓ cup plus 3 tablespoons honey, divided

⅓ cup plus 2 tablespoons canola oil

3 medium eggs

½ teaspoon vanilla extract

Grated zest and juice of 1 medium lemon

1 cup all-purpose flour

½ teaspoon baking soda

¼ teaspoon sea salt

1 cup whipped cream cheese

PER SERVING (1 CUPCAKE): Calories: 253; Fat: 17g; Carbohydrates: 20g; Protein: 7g; Fiber: 1g; Sodium: 188mg; Iron: 1mg

1. Preheat the oven to 350° F. Line a 12-cup muffin tin with muffin liners. Lightly coat each with cooking spray.

2. In a large mixing bowl or stand mixer, combine the ricotta cheese, ⅓ cup plus 2 tablespoons of honey, the oil, eggs, vanilla, 1 teaspoon of lemon zest, and the lemon juice until well mixed.

3. Add the flour, baking soda, and salt. Stir until well incorporated.

4. Fill each prepared muffin cup about three-quarters full (¼ cup of batter).

5. Transfer the muffin tin to the oven and bake for 20 minutes, or until a toothpick inserted into the center of a cupcake comes out clean. Remove from the oven. Place on a wire rack to cool completely.

6. While the cupcakes are baking, in a small bowl, mix together the cream cheese, remaining 1 tablespoon of honey, and 1 teaspoon of lemon zest until smooth. Chill until the cupcakes are completely cool.

7. Frost each cupcake with 1 rounded tablespoon of the cream cheese and honey mixture. Refrigerate leftover frosting and cupcakes in separate airtight containers for up to 4 days.

MAPLE-TAHINI BROWNIES

MAKES 12 SQUARES | **PREP TIME:** 10 MINUTES | **COOK TIME:** 25 MINUTES,
PLUS 15 MINUTES TO COOL

LEFTOVER-FRIENDLY | **NUT-FREE** | **VEGETARIAN**

The mixture of maple and tahini brings these cake-like brownies to a whole new flavor level. It's a great opportunity to use that tahini you may have bought ages ago and aren't sure what to do with, but be aware: tahini can become dry if not mixed well before each use. If yours is too pasty, swap out 1 tablespoon of the tahini for 1 tablespoon of oil.

Nonstick cooking spray, for coating the baking dish (optional)

½ cup tahini

½ cup maple syrup

½ cup chocolate chips, melted

2 medium eggs

½ teaspoon vanilla extract

¼ cup unsweetened cocoa powder

2 tablespoons all-purpose flour

¼ teaspoon sea salt

¼ teaspoon baking powder

PER SERVING (1 SQUARE):
Calories: 161; Fat: 9g; Carbohydrates: 19g; Protein: 3g; Fiber: 2g; Sodium: 31mg; Iron: 1mg

1. Preheat the oven to 350°F. Line a 9-inch square baking dish with parchment paper, or lightly grease it with cooking spray.

2. In a medium bowl, combine the tahini, maple syrup, melted chocolate, eggs, and vanilla until smooth and creamy.

3. Add the cocoa powder, flour, salt, and baking powder. Stir until just combined. Pour into the baking dish.

4. Transfer the baking dish to the oven and bake for 20 to 25 minutes, or until a toothpick inserted into the center of the brownies comes out clean. Place on a wire rack to cool for 15 minutes before cutting into 12 squares. Refrigerate leftover brownies in an airtight container for up to 4 days, or store them at room temperature for up to 2 days.

SUBSTITUTION TIP: Brownies only need a little flour and don't require much leavening. For a gluten-free option that's equally decadent, swap out the flour for 2 tablespoons of almond meal.

MAPLE-SESAME OAT CAKE WITH BLUEBERRY TOPPING

MAKES 1 (8-INCH) CAKE | PREP TIME: 10 MINUTES | **COOK TIME:** 25 MINUTES, PLUS 30 MINUTES TO COOL

LEFTOVER-FRIENDLY | VEGETARIAN

I've always wanted to make an oat cake, and I had a particular idea of what I wanted it to be. After multiple trials, I found this combination of ingredients to be satisfying in both flavor and nutrition. Wild blueberries add an intense punch of flavor to this maple-sweetened treat.

Nonstick cooking spray, for greasing the cake pan

¾ cup unsweetened almond milk

½ cup maple syrup

2 tablespoons tahini

2 medium eggs

2¼ cups rolled oats

¼ cup all-purpose flour

2 tablespoons flax meal

¼ teaspoon sea salt

1 tablespoon apple cider vinegar

1 teaspoon baking soda

1 cup frozen wild blueberries, thawed

PER SERVING (3 OUNCES): Calories: 194; Fat: 8g; Protein: 6g; Carbohydrates: 30g; Fiber: 4g; Sodium: 274mg; Iron: 2mg

1. Preheat the oven to 350°F. Lightly grease an 8-inch round cake pan with cooking spray.

2. In a large bowl, combine the almond milk, maple syrup, tahini, and eggs. Mix until well combined.

3. In a separate large bowl, combine the oats, flour, flax meal, and salt. To make the batter, combine with the wet mixture.

4. Add the vinegar and baking soda. Mix well. (You may see it fizz—that's the chemical reaction that will allow the batter to rise in the oven.) Pour the batter into the prepared cake pan.

5. Transfer the cake pan to the oven and bake for 25 minutes, or until a toothpick inserted into the center of the cake comes out clean. Remove from the oven. Place on a wire rack to cool for 30 minutes.

6. Remove the cake from the pan. Slice into 8 wedges.
7. Serve each slice with 2 tablespoons of wild blueberries (juice included).

INGREDIENT TIP: Wild blueberries have more intensity and antioxidant potential (33 percent more anthocyanins—pigmented antioxidants linked to blood pressure control and anti-inflammatory effects) than ordinary blueberries. You can find frozen wild blueberries at your local grocery store.

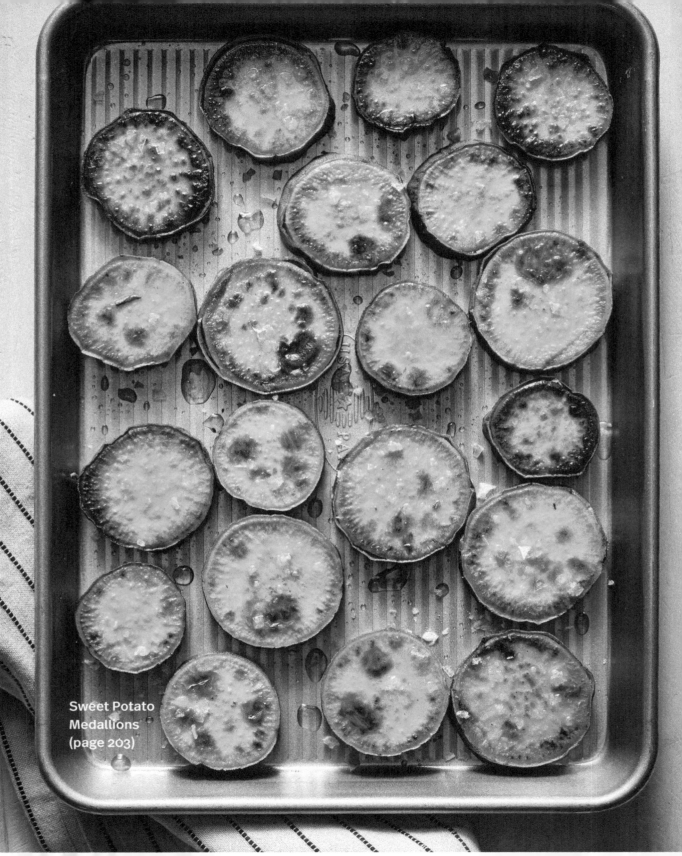

Sweet Potato
Medallions
(page 203)

CHAPTER 10

SNACKS, SIDES, AND STAPLES

Date-Sweetened Teriyaki Sauce **190**

Date-Sweetened Barbecue Sauce **191**

Lemon-Basil Vinaigrette **192**

Sesame Dressing **193**

Creamy Cilantro Dressing **194**

Turmeric-Tahini Dressing **195**

Avocado-Dill Dressing **196**

Lemon-Caper Aïoli **197**

DIY Taco Seasoning **198**

5-Ingredient Mirepoix **199**

Ginger Pickled Radish **200**

Crispy Chickpeas **201**

Kale Crisps **202**

Sweet Potato Medallions **203**

Honey-Glazed Carrots **204**

DATE-SWEETENED TERIYAKI SAUCE

MAKES ¾ CUP | PREP TIME: 5 MINUTES
ONE POT/PAN | LEFTOVER-FRIENDLY | NUT-FREE | VEGAN

This sauce is a thick, creamy flavor enhancer for several recipes in this book, including a variety of bowls and mains. The simple, five-ingredient staple is a quick go-to for flavoring any grain, protein, or starchy veggie. A tablespoon or two is all you need.

2 tablespoons low-sodium soy sauce

1 tablespoon grated peeled fresh ginger root

2 garlic cloves, minced

8 small pitted dates

1 tablespoon apple cider vinegar

⅓ cup water

Put the soy sauce, ginger, garlic, dates, vinegar, and water in a blender. Process until well combined. Transfer to an airtight container and store in the refrigerator for up to a week.

INGREDIENT TIP: For convenience, I often use Dorot Gardens frozen ginger and garlic cubes. For 1 tablespoon ginger root, use 3 cubes; for 2 garlic cloves, use 2 cubes.

**PER SERVING
(2 TABLESPOONS):** Calories: 34; Fat: 0g; Carbohydrates: 8g; Protein: 1g; Fiber: 1g; Sodium: 304mg; Iron: 0mg

DATE-SWEETENED BARBECUE SAUCE

MAKES 1½ CUPS | PREP TIME: 5 MINUTES

ONE POT/PAN | LEFTOVER-FRIENDLY | NUT-FREE | VEGETARIAN

This barbecue sauce is milder than most, making it an ideal choice for families with young kids. I liken it to a more savory and flavorful ketchup. If you prefer the heat, add ¼ teaspoon of chili sauce or Sriracha (a little can go a long way).

⅔ cup tomato paste

⅔ cup low-sodium marinara sauce

2 tablespoons apple cider vinegar

9 small, pitted dates

1 tablespoon honey

½ teaspoon garlic powder

½ teaspoon onion powder

1 teaspoon low-sodium Worcestershire sauce

½ cup water

Put the tomato paste, marinara sauce, vinegar, dates, honey, garlic powder, onion powder, Worcestershire sauce, and water in a blender. Process until well combined. Transfer to an airtight container and store in the refrigerator for up to a week.

PER SERVING (3 TABLESPOONS): Calories: 61; Fat: 0g; Carbohydrates: 14g; Protein: 1g; Fiber: 2g; Sodium: 98mg; Iron: 1mg

LEMON-BASIL VINAIGRETTE

MAKES 1 CUP | PREP TIME: 5 MINUTES

ONE POT/PAN | LEFTOVER-FRIENDLY | GLUTEN-FREE | NUT-FREE | VEGAN

Lemon is the star of this herbal vinaigrette, but basil plays a strong supporting role. This dressing is perfect for any leafy green salad.

½ cup olive oil

½ cup freshly squeezed lemon juice

½ cup chopped fresh basil leaves

2 garlic cloves, minced

½ teaspoon Dijon mustard

2 small, pitted dates

⅛ teaspoon sea salt

PER SERVING (1 TABLESPOON): Calories: 64; Fat: 7g; Carbohydrates: 1g; Protein: 0g; Fiber: 0g; Sodium: 4mg; Iron: 0mg

Put the oil, lemon juice, basil, garlic, mustard, dates, and salt in a blender. Process until well combined. Transfer to an airtight container and store in the refrigerator for up to a week.

SUBSTITUTION TIP: If you don't have Dijon, you can replace it with an equal amount of yellow mustard or a teaspoon of capers.

SESAME DRESSING

MAKES 1 CUP | **PREP TIME:** 5 MINUTES
ONE POT/PAN | **LEFTOVER-FRIENDLY** | **VEGETARIAN**

This dressing departs from the bold flavor profile of the date-sweetened teriyaki sauce, though it's still inspired by Asian cuisine. Tangy yet mildly sweet, this dressing features sesame in two different forms: whole seeds and tahini (which is made from ground sesame seeds). For an even more intense sesame flavor, swap out the canola oil for sesame oil.

¼ cup low-sodium soy sauce

4 teaspoons tahini or all-natural peanut butter

2 tablespoons apple cider vinegar

¼ cup canola oil

1 tablespoon honey

1 to 2 teaspoons grated peeled fresh ginger root

⅓ cup water

1 teaspoon cornstarch

2 teaspoons toasted sesame seeds

1. Put the soy sauce, tahini, vinegar, oil, honey, ginger, water, and cornstarch in a blender. Process until well combined. Transfer to an airtight container.

2. Mix in the sesame seeds and store in the refrigerator for up to a week.

PER SERVING (2 TABLESPOONS): Calories: 94; Fat: 8g; Carbohydrates: 4g; Protein: 1g; Fiber: 0g; Sodium: 296mg; Iron: 0mg

CREAMY CILANTRO DRESSING

MAKES 1½ CUPS | PREP TIME: 5 MINUTES

ONE POT/PAN | LEFTOVER-FRIENDLY | GLUTEN-FREE | NUT-FREE | VEGETARIAN

This is my favorite herb-enhanced dressing. It reminds me of green goddess—a nomenclature I can get behind. It's creamy, refreshing, and mouthwateringly delicious. Toss it on leafy greens, drizzle it on a macro bowl, or use it as a complement to taco-seasoned dishes. It's even a great way to dress up sweet potatoes. There are so many ways to enjoy it!

1 small bunch cilantro (1½ cups loosely packed leaves), coarsely chopped

2 garlic cloves, minced

Juice of 1 lemon

¼ cup canola or sunflower oil

1 cup plain low-fat Greek yogurt

½ teaspoon sea salt

Pinch freshly ground black pepper (optional)

PER SERVING (2 TABLESPOONS): Calories: 59; Fat: 5g; Protein: 3g; Carbohydrates: 2g; Fiber: 0g; Sodium: 107mg; Iron: 0.1mg

In a food processor, combine the cilantro, garlic, lemon juice, oil, yogurt, and salt. Process until smooth and creamy. Add the black pepper (if using). Transfer to an airtight container and store in the refrigerator for up to a week.

VARIATION TIP: The dressing is delicious as is, but you can add 2 minced scallions (green and white parts) and pulse toward the end of processing to add some flecks of texture to your dressing.

TURMERIC–TAHINI DRESSING

MAKES 1⅓ CUPS | PREP TIME: 5 MINUTES

ONE POT/PAN | LEFTOVER-FRIENDLY | GLUTEN-FREE | NUT-FREE | VEGAN

Use this earthy, Mediterranean-inspired condiment to dress up your macro bowls or season your beans and legumes. It's equally delicious on sweet potatoes or as a complement to veggie burgers. Like my creamy cilantro dressing, this one has so many tasty possibilities, making it another staple I keep on hand.

6 small, pitted dates

⅓ cup water, plus ½ cup

½ cup tahini

2 tablespoons ground turmeric

2 tablespoons minced garlic

2 tablespoons apple cider vinegar

Juice of 2 lemons

1 teaspoon sea salt

1 tablespoon canola oil

1. In a blender, combine the dates and ⅓ cup of water. Process to make a paste.

2. Add the tahini, turmeric, garlic, vinegar, lemon juice, salt, and oil. Process until smooth and creamy. Transfer to an airtight container and store in the refrigerator for up to 2 weeks.

**PER SERVING
(2 TABLESPOONS):** Calories: 118; Fat: 10g; Carbohydrates: 5g; Protein: 3g; Fiber: 2g; Sodium: 70mg; Iron: 3mg

AVOCADO-DILL DRESSING

MAKES 1 CUP | PREP TIME: 5 MINUTES

ONE POT/PAN | LEFTOVER-FRIENDLY | GLUTEN-FREE | NUT-FREE | VEGAN

This herb-centric dressing is rich and creamy. It makes for a great alternative to mayonnaise and is perfect for slathering on Avocado-Dill Poached Salmon (page 114) or using as a dip for air-fried sweet potato fries. Use it as a sandwich spread, or mix it with crumbled tofu for a vegan "egg salad." The possibilities are delicious and plentiful.

1¼ medium, ripe avocados, pitted and peeled

3 tablespoons canola oil

2 tablespoons apple cider vinegar

Juice of 2 limes

3 tablespoons freshly squeezed lemon juice

2 tablespoons minced fresh dill

1 garlic clove, minced

3 small, pitted dates

¼ cup water

Put the avocados, oil, vinegar, limes, lemon juice, dill, garlic, dates, and water in a blender. Process until well combined. Transfer to an airtight container and store in the refrigerator for up to a week.

INGREDIENT TIP: If you've got a mini food processor, it's a time-saving, hassle-free way to finely chop herbs such as dill.

PER SERVING (2 TABLESPOONS): Calories: 77; Fat: 8g; Carbohydrates: 2g; Protein: 1g; Fiber: 1g; Sodium: 40mg; Iron: 0mg

LEMON-CAPER AÏOLI

MAKES 1½ CUPS | PREP TIME: 5 MINUTES

ONE POT/PAN | LEFTOVER-FRIENDLY | GLUTEN-FREE | NUT-FREE | VEGETARIAN

This creamy, zesty spread is perfect for sandwiches and burgers and a great way to season your baked fish. It's lower in fat than most aïolis because it substitutes much of the mayonnaise with Greek yogurt.

¼ cup plain low-fat Greek yogurt

3 tablespoons low-fat mayonnaise

4 teaspoons Dijon mustard

2 garlic cloves, minced

Juice of 1 medium lemon

2 teaspoons capers

PER SERVING (2 TABLESPOONS): Calories: 50; Fat: 3g; Carbohydrates: 4g; Protein: 2g; Fiber: 1g; Sodium: 319mg; Iron: 0mg

1. In a blender, combine the yogurt, mayonnaise, mustard, garlic, and lemon juice. Process until smooth and creamy. Transfer to an airtight container.

2. Mix in the capers and store in the refrigerator for up to a week.

TECHNICAL TIP: To simplify the prep, swap out the minced garlic for ½ teaspoon of garlic powder, whisk the ingredients until well combined, and stir in the capers.

DIY TACO SEASONING

MAKES ¾ CUP | PREP TIME: 5 MINUTES

ONE POT/PAN | LEFTOVER-FRIENDLY | GLUTEN-FREE | NUT-FREE | VEGAN

This do-it-yourself blend is great for seasoning all manner of vegetables, beans, meatloaf, veggie burgers, and so much more. Building your own blend ensures that there won't be any of the maltodextrin or cornstarch you'll find in a typical highly processed store-bought mix—just a simple combination of spices that most of us have in our cupboards.

2 tablespoons
   ground cumin

2 tablespoons
   dried oregano

2 tablespoons ground
   cinnamon

¼ cup garlic powder

1 tablespoon sea salt

1 tablespoon cayenne or
   red pepper flakes

PER SERVING (1 TEASPOON):
Calories: 7; Fat: 0g;
Carbohydrates: 2g; Protein:
0g; Fiber: 0g; Sodium: 196mg;
Iron: 0mg

In a small bowl, stir together the cumin, oregano, cinnamon, garlic powder, salt, and cayenne until well combined. Transfer to an airtight jar and store in your cupboard for up to 2 years.

SUBSTITUTION TIP: If you find the heat of cayenne too intense, use just 1 teaspoon and swap out the remaining cayenne for 1 additional teaspoon cumin and 1 additional teaspoon garlic.

5-INGREDIENT MIREPOIX

MAKES 2 CUPS | PREP TIME: 5 MINUTES

LEFTOVER-FRIENDLY | GLUTEN-FREE | NUT-FREE | VEGAN

A traditionally French combination of carrot, onion, and celery, mirepoix carries a deliciously intense and aromatic flavor when cooked. My version is inspired by Italian sofrito, a type of mirepoix that uses a minced veggie blend and olive oil instead of butter. You'll use this blend as a base for lots of different main dishes.

1 to 2 teaspoons olive oil

5 medium white or cremini mushrooms, minced

1 cup minced yellow onion

1 medium carrot, minced

1 medium celery stalk, minced

Cook according to the method in the primary recipe, or refrigerate in an airtight container for later use.

VARIATION TIP: If you have chronic acid reflux (GERD) or any other digestive condition for which onion is a trigger, swap it out for an equal amount of minced fennel bulb.

PER SERVING (2 TABLESPOONS): Calories: 15; Fat: 1g; Carbohydrates: 2g; Protein: 0g; Fiber: 0g; Sodium: 6mg; Iron: 0mg

GINGER PICKLED RADISH

MAKES ⅔ CUP | PREP TIME: 5 MINUTES (PLUS 3 TO 5 DAYS TO CURE)

ONE POT/PAN | LEFTOVER-FRIENDLY | GLUTEN-FREE | NUT-FREE | VEGAN

Crisp and tangy, these radish pickles are a perfect complement to salads and bowls. They're also a great alternative to the typical pickled cucumber in sandwiches and wraps. Note: These pickles take at least a few days to cure, so be sure to prepare a batch in advance if you are looking forward to including this amazing garnish in your meals.

⅔ cup thinly sliced radish

3 garlic cloves, minced

1 tablespoon grated peeled fresh ginger root

½ cup apple cider vinegar

½ cup water

PER SERVING (1 TABLESPOON SLICED PICKLED RADISH): Calories: 4; Fat: 0g; Carbohydrates: 1g; Protein: 0g; Fiber: 0g; Sodium: 5mg; Iron: 0mg

In a jar, combine the radish, garlic, ginger, vinegar, and water. Seal tightly and refrigerate for at least 3 days before using.

TECHNICAL TIP: Avoid the temptation to cut your garlic and ginger into large pieces. Because they all turn pink in the pickling liquid, it's too easy to confuse a whole garlic clove for a radish, which makes for quite a surprise when you pop one in your mouth!

CRISPY CHICKPEAS

MAKES ABOUT 1 CUP | **PREP TIME:** 5 MINUTES | **COOK TIME:** 25 MINUTES

LEFTOVER-FRIENDLY | **GLUTEN-FREE** | **NUT-FREE** | **VEGAN**

Roasted chickpeas are a perfect alternative to croutons, nuts, and other crunchy toppings. Part of the legume family, chickpeas provide the benefits of protein and fiber, and they also contain resistant starch, which helps balance blood sugars and make probiotics (found in yogurt, kefir, and sauerkraut) more effective.

1 (14-ounce) can low-sodium chickpeas, drained and rinsed

2 teaspoons olive oil or canola oil

½ teaspoon sea salt

PER SERVING (3 TABLESPOONS): Calories: 80; Fat: 3g; Carbohydrates: 10g; Protein: 3g; Fiber: 3g; Sodium: 158mg; Iron: 1mg

1. Preheat the oven to 400°F.
2. Using a paper towel, thoroughly dry the chickpeas to remove most of the excess water (or spin in a salad spinner). Dried chickpeas will result in a crispier texture.
3. In a large, resealable plastic bag, combine the chickpeas, oil, and salt. Seal and shake vigorously to thoroughly coat. Pour onto a baking tray.
4. Transfer the baking tray to the oven and bake for 25 minutes, stirring after 15 minutes, or until the chickpeas are thoroughly toasted and crisp. Remove from the oven.

VARIATION TIP: Try adding 1 teaspoon cinnamon for a slightly more complex flavor.

KALE CRISPS

SERVES 4 | **PREP TIME:** 5 MINUTES | **COOK TIME:** 15 MINUTES

GLUTEN-FREE | **NUT-FREE** | **VEGAN**

I love the simplicity of making this crispy snack. You'll want to thoroughly coat your kale with oil and salt so that each leaf is well seasoned before baking (a sealable plastic bag does the trick). Then it's just a matter of popping the kale in the oven to crisp.

5 cups chopped
    lacinato kale

2 teaspoons olive oil

⅛ teaspoon sea salt

½ teaspoon garlic powder

PER SERVING (¼ BATCH):
Calories: 53; Fat: 3g;
Carbohydrates: 7g; Protein:
2g; Fiber: 2g; Sodium: 98mg;
Iron: 1mg

1. Preheat the oven to 350°F.
2. In a large, resealable plastic bag, combine the kale, oil, salt, and garlic powder. Seal and shake well until the kale is completely coated. Massage the bag if needed to tenderize the kale further.
3. Lay out the seasoned kale in 1 even layer on a large baking sheet.
4. Transfer the baking sheet to the oven and bake for 12 minutes, or until the kale is crisp. If not all pieces are crisp, turn off the oven and use a spatula to turn over the kale pieces. Leave them in the residual heat of the oven for a few more minutes until they are crispy.

INGREDIENT TIP: For a fun flavor addition, add 1 ounce grated parmesan to the plastic bag with the other ingredients. Shake well and bake.

SWEET POTATO MEDALLIONS

SERVES 4 | PREP TIME: 5 MINUTES **| COOK TIME:** 40 MINUTES

LEFTOVER-FRIENDLY | GLUTEN-FREE | NUT-FREE | VEGAN

Because sweet potatoes are so versatile, the recipe here is pretty neutral, adding just enough flavor but no strong savory or sweet influences. That means you can enjoy the potatoes alone or tailor them to fit within your desired craving—be it teriyaki, cinnamon, or Creamy Cilantro Dressing (page 194).

3 medium sweet potatoes, thickly sliced

2 teaspoons olive oil or canola oil

⅛ teaspoon sea salt

1 tablespoon chopped fresh basil leaves (optional)

PER SERVING (3 TABLESPOONS): Calories: 103; Fat: 2g; Carbohydrates: 0g; Protein: 2g; Fiber: 3g; Sodium: 20mg; Iron: 1mg

1. Preheat the oven to 400°F. Line a large baking sheet with aluminum foil.

2. In a sealable plastic bag, combine the sweet potatoes, oil, and salt. Seal and shake vigorously to thoroughly coat. Transfer to the prepared baking sheet in 1 layer.

3. Transfer the baking sheet to the oven and roast for 30 to 40 minutes, or until the sweet potatoes are tender. Remove from the oven.

4. Garnish with the basil (if using). Refrigerate in an airtight container for up to 4 days.

TECHNICAL TIP: Roast these sweet potatoes under a rack holding chicken, pork, or beef so the juices drip over them and caramelize as they bake.

HONEY-GLAZED CARROTS

SERVES 4 | **PREP TIME:** 5 MINUTES | **COOK TIME:** 20 MINUTES

ONE POT/PAN | **LEFTOVER-FRIENDLY** | **GLUTEN-FREE** | **NUT-FREE** | **VEGETARIAN**

These honey-sweetened carrots come together deliciously in this easy skillet recipe. To complement the honey's sweetness and add some color to the dish, garnish the carrots with finely chopped basil, mint, or cilantro.

1 tablespoon canola oil

7 medium carrots, thickly sliced

½ cup water

⅛ teaspoon sea salt

1 tablespoon honey

¼ teaspoon ground cinnamon

PER SERVING (¼ OF THE BATCH): Calories: 82; Fat: 4g; Carbohydrates: 13g; Protein: 1g; Fiber: 3g; Sodium: 133mg; Iron: 0mg

1. In a medium skillet, heat the oil over medium heat for 30 seconds, or until shimmering.

2. Add the carrots, water, salt, and honey. Stir to coat. Cover the skillet and heat for 10 minutes, or until the carrots begin to soften.

3. Reduce the heat to low. Cook for 10 minutes, or until the carrots are tender. Remove from the heat.

4. Dust with the cinnamon and serve. Refrigerate leftovers in an airtight container for up to 5 days.

MEASUREMENT CONVERSIONS

VOLUME EQUIVALENTS	U.S. STANDARD	U.S. STANDARD (OUNCES)	METRIC (APPROXIMATE)
LIQUID	2 tablespoons	1 fl. oz.	30 mL
	¼ cup	2 fl. oz.	60 mL
	½ cup	4 fl. oz.	120 mL
	1 cup	8 fl. oz.	240 mL
	1½ cups	12 fl. oz.	355 mL
	2 cups or 1 pint	16 fl. oz.	475 mL
	4 cups or 1 quart	32 fl. oz.	1 L
	1 gallon	128 fl. oz.	4 L
DRY	⅛ teaspoon		0.5 mL
	¼ teaspoon		1 mL
	½ teaspoon		2 mL
	¾ teaspoon		4 mL
	1 teaspoon		5 mL
	1 tablespoon		15 mL
	¼ cup		59 mL
	⅓ cup		79 mL
	½ cup		118 mL
	⅔ cup		156 mL
	¾ cup		177 mL
	1 cup		235 mL
	2 cups or 1 pint		475 mL
	3 cups		700 mL
	4 cups or 1 quart		1 L
	½ gallon		2 L
	1 gallon		4 L

OVEN TEMPERATURES

FAHRENHEIT	CELSIUS (APPROXIMATE)
250°F	120°C
300°F	150°C
325°F	165°C
350°F	180°C
375°F	190°C
400°F	200°C
425°F	220°C
450°F	230°C

WEIGHT EQUIVALENTS

U.S. STANDARD	METRIC (APPROXIMATE)
½ ounce	15 g
1 ounce	30 g
2 ounces	60 g
4 ounces	115 g
8 ounces	225 g
12 ounces	340 g
16 ounces or 1 pound	455 g

RESOURCES

Anti-Inflammatory Diet Meal Prep: 6 Weekly Plans and 80+ Recipes to Simplify Your Healing

By Ginger Hultin, MS, RDN, CSO

This book will help you prepare delicious, healing, portion-controlled meals. You'll learn how to prep ahead to have ready-to-eat meals at your convenience.

Clean Eating for Busy Families: Get Meals on the Table in Minutes with Simple and Satisfying Whole-Foods Recipes You and Your Kids Will Love— Most Recipes Take Just 30 Minutes or Less!

By Michelle Dudash, RD

With a focus on whole foods, this family-friendly cookbook keeps it simple, tasty, and doable to get healthy meals on the table every day.

Healthy Smoothie Recipe Book: Easy Mix-and-Match Smoothie Recipes for a Healthier You

By Jennifer Koslo, PhD, RD, CSSD

Provides more than 100 recipes for easy-to-make, nutritious smoothies with customizable options and troubleshooting tips.

The Complete Anti-Inflammatory Diet for Beginners: A No-Stress Meal Plan with Easy Recipes to Heal the Immune System

By Dorothy Calimeris and Lulu Cook

A no-nonsense anti-inflammatory dietary guide with simple, tasty recipes for improved health and healing.

The Mediterranean DASH Diet Cookbook: Lower Your Blood Pressure and Improve Your Health

By Abbie Gellman, CDN, MS, RD

This cookbook combines two of the most consistently recommended, evidence-based diets for improved health. It contains 100 delicious, easy-to-make, plant-based recipes.

REFERENCES

Academy of Nutrition and Dietetics. "Sugar Substitutes: How Much Is Too Much?" *Eat Right* (blog).
Accessed March 13, 2021. EatRight.org/food/nutrition/dietary-guidelines-and-myplate
/sugar-substitutes-how-much-is-too-much.

Çakmur, Hülya. "Introductory Chapter: How Does Stress Impact Human Body?" In *Effects of Stress on Human Health*. IntechOpen, 2020. DOI.org/10.5772/intechopen.91984.

Choudhary, Arbind Kumar. "Aspartame: Should Individuals with Type II Diabetes Be Taking It?"
Current Diabetes Reviews 14, no. 4 (2018): 350–62. DOI.org/10.2174/1573399813666170601093336.

Derbyshire, Emma. "Brain Health across the Lifespan: A Systematic Review on the Role of Omega-3
Fatty Acid Supplements." *Nutrients* 10, no. 8 (2018): 1094. DOI.org/10.3390/nu10081094.

Dietary Guidelines for Americans. "Home: Dietary Guidelines for Americans." Accessed February 16,
2021. DietaryGuidelines.gov.

DiNicolantonio, James J., Sean C. Lucan, and James H. O'Keefe. "The Evidence for Saturated Fat and
for Sugar Related to Coronary Heart Disease." *Progress in Cardiovascular Diseases* 58, no. 5 (2016):
464–72. DOI.org/10.1016/j.pcad.2015.11.006.

Duan, Lihua, Xiaoquan Rao, and Keshav Raj Sigdel. "Regulation of Inflammation in Autoimmune
Disease." *Journal of Immunology Research* 2019 (2019). DOI.org/10.1155/2019/7403796.

Ebbeling, Cara B., Ian S. Young, Alice H. Lichtenstein, David S. Ludwig, Michelle McKinley, Rafael
Perez-Escamilla, and Eric Rimm. "Dietary Fat: Friend or Foe?" *Clinical Chemistry* 64, no. 1 (January
2018): 34–41. DOI.org/10.1373/clinchem.2017.274084.

Gutiérrez, Saray, Sara L. Svahn, and Maria E. Johansson. "Effects of Omega-3 Fatty Acids on Immune
Cells." *International Journal of Molecular Sciences* 20, no. 20 (2019): 5028. DOI.org/10.3390
/ijms20205028.

Hibi, Masanobu, Chie Kubota, Tomohito Mizuno, Sayaka Aritake, Yuki Mitsui, Mitsuhiro Katashima,
and Sunao Uchida. "Effect of Shortened Sleep on Energy Expenditure, Core Body Temperature, and Appetite: A Human Randomised Crossover Trial." *Scientific Reports* 7 (2017): 39640.
DOI.org/10.1038/srep39640.

López-Candales, Angel, and David Harris. "From Bench to Bedside: Chronic Inflammation and
Cardiovascular Risks." *IJC Metabolic & Endocrine* 12 (September 2016): 1–2. DOI.org/10.1016
/j.ijcme.2016.05.004.

Mayo Clinic. "Water: How Much Should You Drink Every Day?" October 14, 2020. MayoClinic.org /healthy-lifestyle/nutrition-and-healthy-eating/in-depth/water/art-20044256.

Mualem, Raed, Gerry Leisman, Yusra Zbedat, Sherif Ganem, Ola Mualem, Monjed Amaria, Aiman Kozle, Safa Khayat-Moughrabi, and Alon Ornai. "The Effect of Movement on Cognitive Performance." *Frontiers in Public Health* 6 (2018): 100. DOI.org/10.3389/fpubh.2018.00100.

Nettleton, Jodi E., Raylene A. Reimer, and Jane Shearer. "Reshaping the Gut Microbiota: Impact of Low Calorie Sweeteners and the Link to Insulin Resistance?" *Physiology and Behavior* 164 (2016): 488–93. DOI.org/10.1016/j.physbeh.2016.04.029.

Popkin, Barry M., Kristen E. D'Anci, and Irwin H. Rosenberg. "Water, Hydration, and Health." *Nutrition Reviews* 68, no. 8 (2010): 439–58. DOI.org/10.1111/j.1753-4887.2010.00304.x.

Purohit, Vikas, and Sundeep Mishra. "The Truth about Artificial Sweeteners—Are They Good for Diabetics?" *Indian Heart Journal* 70, no. 1 (2018): 197–99. DOI.org/10.1016/j.ihj.2018.01.020.

"Rat Brain Fatty Acids in Essential Fatty Acid Deficiency." *Nutrition Reviews* 30, no. 1 (January 1972): 18–21. DOI.org/10.1111/j.1753-4887.1972.tb03972.x.

Skonieczna-Żydecka, Karolina, Wojciech Marlicz, Agata Misera, Anastasios Koulaouzidis, and Igor Łoniewski. "Microbiome—The Missing Link in the Gut-Brain Axis: Focus on Its Role in Gastrointestinal and Mental Health." *Journal of Clinical Medicine* 7, no. 12 (2018): 521. DOI.org/10.3390/jcm7120521.

World Health Organization. "Physical Activity." Accessed February 16, 2021. WHO.int/news-room /fact-sheets/detail/physical-activity.

Yang, Quanhe, Zefeng Zhang, Edward W. Gregg, W. Dana Flanders, Robert Merritt, and Frank B. Hu. "Added Sugar Intake and Cardiovascular Diseases Mortality among US Adults." *JAMA Internal Medicine* 174, no. 4 (2014): 516–24. DOI.org/10.1001/jamainternmed.2013.13563.

Yaribeygi, Habib, Yunes Panahi, Hedayat Sahraei, Thomas P. Johnston, and Amirhossein Sahebkar. "The Impact of Stress on Body Function: A Review." *EXCLI Journal* 16 (2017): 1057–72. DOI.org/10.17179/excli2017-480.

INDEX

A

Aïoli
  Lemon-Caper Aïoli, 197
  Tuna Toasts with Lemon-Caper Aïoli, 96
Almonds
  Coconut-Almond Macaroons, 182–183
  Honey-Almond Energy Bites, 180
Apples
  Apple and Walnut Salad over Greens, 62
  Apple Flapjacks, 48
  Turkey, Apple, and Cranberry Meatballs, 142–143
Arugula Salad, Shrimp and, 98
Asparagus Soup, Cream of, 58
Autoimmune disorders, 6
Avocados
  Avocado-Dill Dressing, 196
  Avocado-Dill Poached Salmon, 114–115
  Blueberry-Basil Avocado Toasts, 34
  Chickpea, Lentil, and Avocado Sandwiches, 63
  Chocolate-Avocado Pudding, 178
  Sesame Avocado Salad, 57
  Sesame Avocado Salad with Tuna, 97

B

Balanced plate, 2–3
Banana-Nut Overnight Oats, 36
Barbecue
  Barbecue-Glazed Meatloaf, 162–163
  Barbecue Pork Chops, 152–153
  Barbecue Turkey Bowls, 146–147
  Date-Sweetened Barbecue Sauce, 191
Basil
  Blueberry-Basil Avocado Toasts, 34
  Cucumber, Tomato, and Basil Salad, 60
  Lemon-Basil Vinaigrette, 192
  Lentil "Meat"balls with Basil and Parmesan, 70–71
  Strawberry-Basil Smoothie, 41
  Strawberry-Spinach Salad with
    Lemon-Basil Vinaigrette, 61
Beans
  Black Bean Fiesta Bowls, 80
  Spaghetti and Vegetarian "Meat"balls, 92–93
  Teriyaki Black Bean Burgers, 72–73

Beef
  Barbecue-Glazed Meatloaf, 162–163
  Beef and Broccoli Stir-Fry, 166–167
  Beef and Mushroom Burgers, 164–165
  Grilled Rosemary Flank Steak with
    Seasoned Farro, 170–171
  Lightened Beef Stroganoff, 172–173
  Peppered Beef Macro Bowls, 168
  Steak Salad with Sesame Dressing, 169
  Stuffed Bell Peppers, 160–161
Bell peppers
  Mexican-Inspired Tilapia with Bell
    Peppers and Kale, 106
  Pan-Seared Pork Chops with Kale,
    Corn, and Bell Pepper, 154–155
  Sautéed Eggplant with Peppers and Onions, 75
  Stuffed Bell Peppers, 160–161
Berries
  Blueberry-Basil Avocado Toasts, 34
  Blueberry-Peach Smoothie, 44
  Lemon-Blueberry Parfaits, 176
  Maple-Sesame Oat Cake with
    Blueberry Topping, 186–187
  Strawberries and Cream, 179
  Strawberry-Basil Smoothie, 41
  Strawberry-Spinach Salad with
    Lemon-Basil Vinaigrette, 61
  Turkey, Apple, and Cranberry Meatballs, 142–143
Black Bean Fiesta Bowls, 80
Blueberries
  Blueberry-Basil Avocado Toasts, 34
  Blueberry-Peach Smoothie, 44
  Lemon-Blueberry Parfaits, 176
  Maple-Sesame Oat Cake with
    Blueberry Topping, 186–187
Bowls
  Barbecue Turkey Bowls, 146–147
  Black Bean Fiesta Bowls, 80
  Chickpea, Kale, and Sweet Potato
    Bowls, 78
  Fiesta Chicken Macro Bowls, 124–125
  Ginger-Soy Noodle Bowls, 82
  Mediterranean Bowls, 79

Peppered Beef Macro Bowls, 168
Quinoa Harvest Bowls, 81
Sesame Salmon Protein Bowls, 116–117
Spicy Chili Pork Bowls, 156
Teriyaki Salmon Bowls, 113
Breakfasts. See also Smoothies
    Apple Flapjacks, 48
    Banana-Nut Overnight Oats, 36
    Blueberry-Basil Avocado Toasts, 34
    Cinnamon Toast Oatmeal, 35
    Maple-Date Granola, 40
    Pear, Spinach, and Ricotta
        Omelet, 38–39
    Tamale-Style Grits and Eggs, 37
Broccoli Stir-Fry, Beef and, 166–167
Brownies, Maple-Tahini, 185
Burgers and patties
    Beef and Mushroom Burgers, 164–165
    Teriyaki Black Bean Burgers, 72–73
    Turkey Burgers with Creamy
        Cilantro Dressing, 140–141
    Veggie Burger Parmesan, 84–85
Butternut Squash and Tomato Soup, 52

C

Cake with Blueberry Topping, Maple-
    Sesame Oat, 186–187
Capers
    Lemon-Caper Aïoli, 197
    Tuna Toasts with Lemon-Caper
        Aïoli, 96
Carbohydrates, 9
Carrots
    Carrot-Ginger Soup, 55
    Carrot, Mango, and Citrus Smoothie, 45
    5-Ingredient Mirepoix, 199
    Honey-Glazed Carrots, 204
Cashew Chicken, 121
Cauliflower Soup, Curried, 56
Cheese
    Cheesecake Parfaits, 177
    Chicken Parmesan, 136–137
    Lemon-Ricotta Cupcakes, 184
    Lentil "Meat"balls with Basil and Parmesan, 70–71
    Pan-Seared Tilapia over
        Lemon-Parmesan Pasta, 104–105
    Pear, Spinach, and Ricotta Omelet, 38–39
    Roasted Veggie Mac-n-Cheese Au Gratin, 90–91

Veggie Burger Parmesan, 84–85
Cheesecake Parfaits, 177
Chicken, 11
    Cashew Chicken, 121
    Chicken, Lettuce, and Tomato Sandwiches
        with Creamy Cilantro Dressing, 65
    Chicken Parmesan, 136–137
    Dijon Roasted Chicken with Grits, 132–133
    Fiesta Chicken Macro Bowls, 124–125
    Herbed Chicken with Couscous
        and Spinach, 122–123
    One-Pot Chicken with Penne and Tomatoes, 138
    Panko-Crusted Chicken with Dipping
        Sauce Trio, 128–129
    Pineapple Chicken, 126–127
    Sesame Chicken Chopped Salad, 120
    Simple Baked Chicken with Potato and
        Green Bean Salad, 130–131
    Teriyaki Chicken with Kale Salad and
        Sweet Potato Medallions, 134–135
Chickpeas
    Chickpea, Kale, and Sweet Potato Bowls, 78
    Chickpea, Lentil, and Avocado Sandwiches, 63
    Crispy Chickpeas, 201
Chocolate
    Chocolate-Avocado Pudding, 178
    Peanut Butter and Chocolate Chip Cookies, 181
Cilantro
    Baked Salmon with Creamy Cilantro
        Dressing, 112
    Chicken, Lettuce, and Tomato Sandwiches
        with Creamy Cilantro Dressing, 65
    Creamy Cilantro Dressing, 194
    Turkey Burgers with Creamy
        Cilantro Dressing, 140–141
Cinnamon
    Cinnamon Oat and Pear Smoothie, 46
    Cinnamon Toast Oatmeal, 35
Coconut
    Coconut-Almond Macaroons, 182–183
    Coconut-Mango Green Smoothie, 47
Collard Greens, Shrimp and Grits over, 100–101
Cookies
    Coconut-Almond Macaroons, 182–183
    Peanut Butter and Chocolate Chip
        Cookies, 181
Corn, and Bell Pepper, Pan-Seared Pork
    Chops with Kale, 154–155

Couscous
  Herbed Chicken with Couscous
    and Spinach, 122–123
  Italian Wedding Soup, 144–145
Cranberry Meatballs, Turkey, Apple, and, 142–143
Cucumber, Tomato, and Basil Salad, 60
Cupcakes, Lemon-Ricotta, 184
Curried Cauliflower Soup, 54
Curried Lentil Stew, 83

D

Dairy products, 10
Dates
  Date-Sweetened Barbecue Sauce, 191
  Date-Sweetened Teriyaki Sauce, 190
  Maple-Date Granola, 40
Desserts
  Cheesecake Parfaits, 177
  Chocolate-Avocado Pudding, 178
  Coconut-Almond Macaroons, 182–183
  Honey-Almond Energy Bites, 180
  Lemon-Blueberry Parfaits, 176
  Lemon-Ricotta Cupcakes, 184
  Maple-Sesame Oat Cake with
    Blueberry Topping, 186–187
  Maple-Tahini Brownies, 185
  Peanut Butter and Chocolate Chip
    Cookies, 181
  Strawberries and Cream, 179
"Diet" foods, 12–13
Dijon Roasted Chicken with Grits, 132–133
Dill
  Avocado-Dill Dressing, 196
  Avocado-Dill Poached Salmon, 114–115
Dressings
  Avocado-Dill Dressing, 196
  Creamy Cilantro Dressing, 194
  Lemon-Basil Vinaigrette, 192
  Sesame Dressing, 193
  Turmeric-Tahini Dressing, 195

E

Edamame Salad, Sesame Mandarin and, 61
Eggplants
  Sautéed Eggplant with Peppers and Onions, 75
  Stuffed Eggplant with Savory Vegan
    Cream, 76–77

Eggs
  Pear, Spinach, and Ricotta Omelet, 38–39
  Tamale-Style Grits and Eggs, 37
Energy, 7
Exercise, 4

F

Farro
  Grilled Rosemary Flank Steak with
    Seasoned Farro, 170–171
  Tabbouleh Salad with Farro, 58
Fats, 8, 11
Fiber, 6, 9
Fish and seafood, 11
  Avocado-Dill Poached Salmon, 114–115
  Baked Salmon with Creamy Cilantro
    Dressing, 112
  Foil-Wrapped Tuscan Haddock, 107
  Haddock with Creamy Yogurt
    Mayonnaise, 108–109
  Mexican-Inspired Tilapia with Bell
    Peppers and Kale, 106
  One-Pot Taco Shrimp, 99
  Pan-Seared Tilapia over Lemon-
    Parmesan Pasta, 104–105
  Seared Fish Tacos with Mango-Lime
    Salsa, 102–103
  Sesame Avocado Salad with Tuna, 97
  Sesame Salmon Protein Bowls, 116–117
  Shrimp and Arugula Salad, 98
  Shrimp and Grits over Collard Greens, 100–101
  Tahini Roasted Salmon with Warm
    Kale Salad, 110–111
  Teriyaki Salmon Bowls, 113
  Tuna Toasts with Lemon-Caper Aïoli, 96
Flapjacks, Apple, 40–41
Fruits, 10. See also specific

G

Ginger
  Carrot-Ginger Soup, 55
  Ginger Pickled Radish, 200
  Ginger-Soy Noodle Bowls, 82
Gluten-free
  Apple and Walnut Salad over Greens, 62
  Avocado-Dill Dressing, 196
  Baked Salmon with Creamy Cilantro Dressing, 112

Banana-Nut Overnight Oats, 36
Blueberry-Peach Smoothie, 44
Butternut Squash and Tomato Soup, 52
Carrot-Ginger Soup, 55
Carrot, Mango, and Citrus Smoothie, 45
Chocolate-Avocado Pudding, 178
Cinnamon Oat and Pear Smoothie, 46
Cinnamon Toast Oatmeal, 35
Coconut-Almond Macaroons, 182–183
Coconut-Mango Green Smoothie, 47
Cream of Asparagus Soup, 56
Creamy Cilantro Dressing, 194
Crispy Chickpeas, 201
Cucumber, Tomato, and Basil Salad, 60
DIY Taco Seasoning, 198
Fiesta Chicken Macro Bowls, 124–125
5-Ingredient Mirepoix, 199
Foil-Wrapped Tuscan Haddock, 107
Ginger Pickled Radish, 200
Green-Powered Smoothie, 42
Haddock with Creamy Yogurt Mayonnaise, 108–109
Honey-Glazed Carrots, 204
Kale Crisps, 202
Lemon-Basil Vinaigrette, 192
Lemon-Caper Aïoli, 197
Lemony Lentil Soup, 53
Mango Cream Smoothie, 43
Mexican-Inspired Tilapia with Bell
    Peppers and Kale, 106
Pan-Seared Pork Chops with Kale,
    Corn, and Bell Pepper, 154–155
Pear, Spinach, and Ricotta Omelet, 38–39
Peppered Beef Macro Bowls, 168
Quinoa Harvest Bowls, 81
Sautéed Eggplant with Peppers and Onions, 75
Seared Fish Tacos with Mango-Lime
    Salsa, 102–103
Shrimp and Arugula Salad, 98
Shrimp and Grits over Collard Greens, 100–101
Spicy Chili Pork Bowls, 156
Strawberries and Cream, 179
Strawberry-Basil Smoothie, 41
Strawberry-Spinach Salad with
    Lemon-Basil Vinaigrette, 61
Stuffed Eggplant with Savory Vegan Cream, 76–77
Sweet Potato Medallions, 203
Tamale-Style Grits and Eggs, 37

Turmeric-Tahini Dressing, 195
Granola, 13
    Maple-Date Granola, 40
Green Bean Salad, Simple Baked Chicken
    with Potato and, 130–131
Grits
    Dijon Roasted Chicken with Grits, 132–133
    Shrimp and Grits over Collard Greens, 100–101
    Tamale-Style Grits and Eggs, 37
Gut health, 6

H

Haddock
    Foil-Wrapped Tuscan Haddock, 107
    Haddock with Creamy Yogurt
        Mayonnaise, 108–109
Healthy eating
    food categories, 7–9
    foods to eat/limit/avoid, 10–11
    health benefits, 6–7
    rules, 2–3
    tips, 15–16
Herbed Chicken with Couscous and
    Spinach, 122–123
Honey, 11
    Honey-Almond Energy Bites, 180
    Honey-Glazed Carrots, 204
    Honey-Glazed Pork Chops, 150–151
Hummus Tabbouleh Wraps, 64
Hydration, 4

I

Inflammation, 6

K

Kale
    Chickpea, Kale, and Sweet Potato
        Bowls, 78
    Kale Crisps, 202
    Mexican-Inspired Tilapia with Bell
        Peppers and Kale, 106
    Pan-Seared Pork Chops with Kale,
        Corn, and Bell Pepper, 154–155
    Tahini Roasted Salmon with Warm
        Kale Salad, 110–111
    Teriyaki Chicken with Kale Salad and
        Sweet Potato Medallions, 134–135

L

Leftover-friendly

Apple Flapjacks, 48

Avocado-Dill Dressing, 196

Avocado-Dill Poached Salmon, 114–115

Baked Salmon with Creamy Cilantro
    Dressing, 112

Barbecue-Glazed Meatloaf, 162–163

Barbecue Pork Chops, 152–153

Barbecue Turkey Bowls, 146–147

Beef and Broccoli Stir-Fry, 166–167

Butternut Squash and Tomato Soup, 52

Carrot-Ginger Soup, 55

Cashew Chicken, 121

Chicken Parmesan, 136–137

Chickpea, Kale, and Sweet Potato Bowls, 78

Cinnamon Toast Oatmeal, 35

Cream of Asparagus Soup, 56

Creamy Cilantro Dressing, 194

Crispy Chickpeas, 201

Curried Cauliflower Soup, 54

Curried Lentil Stew, 83

Date-Sweetened Barbecue Sauce, 191

Date-Sweetened Teriyaki Sauce, 190

Dijon Roasted Chicken with Grits, 132–133

DIY Taco Seasoning, 198

Fiesta Chicken Macro Bowls, 124–125

5-Ingredient Mirepoix, 199

Foil-Wrapped Tuscan Haddock, 107

Ginger Pickled Radish, 200

Ginger-Soy Noodle Bowls, 82

Grilled Rosemary Flank Steak with
    Seasoned Farro, 170–171

Haddock with Creamy Yogurt Mayonnaise, 108–109

Herbed Chicken with Couscous
    and Spinach, 122–123

Honey-Almond Energy Bites, 180

Honey-Glazed Carrots, 204

Honey-Glazed Pork Chops, 150–151

Italian Wedding Soup, 144–145

Lemon-Basil Vinaigrette, 192

Lemon-Caper Aïoli, 197

Lemon-Ricotta Cupcakes, 184

Lemony Lentil Soup, 53

Lentil "Meat"balls with Basil and Parmesan, 70–71

Lightened Beef Stroganoff, 172–173

Maple-Sesame Oat Cake with
    Blueberry Topping, 186–187

Maple-Tahini Brownies, 185

One-Pot Chicken with Penne and Tomatoes, 138

One-Pot Pasta with Ground Turkey
    and Mushroom Sauce, 139

Panko-Crusted Chicken with Dipping
    Sauce Trio, 128–129

Pan-Seared Pork Chops with Kale,
    Corn, and Bell Pepper, 154–155

Peanut Butter and Chocolate Chip Cookies, 181

Peppered Beef Macro Bowls, 168

Pineapple Chicken, 126–127

Pineapple Pork with Roasted
    Vegetables, 158–159

Quinoa Harvest Bowls, 81

Roasted Veggie Mac-n-Cheese Au Gratin, 90–91

Sautéed Eggplant with Peppers and Onions, 75

Seared Fish Tacos with Mango-Lime
    Salsa, 102–103

Sesame Dressing, 193

Sesame Salmon Protein Bowls, 116–117

Shrimp and Arugula Salad, 98

Simple Baked Chicken with Potato and
    Green Bean Salad, 130–131

Smooth Zucchini Soup, 66

Spaghetti and Vegetarian "Meat"balls, 92–93

Spicy Chili Pork Bowls, 156

Steak Salad with Sesame Dressing, 169

Strawberries and Cream, 179

Stuffed Bell Peppers, 160–161

Stuffed Eggplant with Savory Vegan Cream, 76–77

Sweet Potato Medallions, 203

Tabbouleh Salad with Farro, 58

Tahini Roasted Salmon with Warm
    Kale Salad, 110–111

Tamale-Style Grits and Eggs, 37

Teriyaki Black Bean Burgers, 72–73

Teriyaki Chicken with Kale Salad and
    Sweet Potato Medallions, 134–135

Teriyaki Pork Stir-Fry, 157

Teriyaki Salmon Bowls, 113

Tuna Toasts with Lemon-Caper Aïoli, 96

Turmeric-Tahini Dressing, 195

Vegetarian Shepherd's Pie, 88–89

Veggie Burger Parmesan, 84–85

Veggie Meatloaf, 86–87

Legumes, 10. *See also specific*
Lemons
    Lemon-Basil Vinaigrette, 192
    Lemon-Blueberry Parfaits, 176
    Lemon-Caper Aïoli, 197
    Lemon-Ricotta Cupcakes, 184
    Lemony Lentil Soup, 53
    Pan-Seared Tilapia over Lemon-
        Parmesan Pasta, 104–105
    Strawberry-Spinach Salad with
        Lemon-Basil Vinaigrette, 61
    Tuna Toasts with Lemon-Caper Aïoli, 96
Lentils
    Chickpea, Lentil, and Avocado Sandwiches, 63
    Curried Lentil Stew, 83
    Lemony Lentil Soup, 53
    Lentil "Meat"balls with Basil and Parmesan, 70–71
    Vegetarian Shepherd's Pie, 88–89
Lettuce
    Apple and Walnut Salad over Greens, 62
    Chicken, Lettuce, and Tomato Sandwiches
        with Creamy Cilantro Dressing, 65
Lifestyle changes, 4–5
Lime Salsa, Seared Fish Tacos with Mango-, 102–103

M

Mangos
    Carrot, Mango, and Citrus Smoothie, 45
    Coconut-Mango Green Smoothie, 47
    Mango Cream Smoothie, 43
    Seared Fish Tacos with Mango-Lime
        Salsa, 102–103
Maple syrup, 11
    Maple-Date Granola, 40
    Maple-Sesame Oat Cake with
        Blueberry Topping, 186–187
    Maple-Tahini Brownies, 185
Mayonnaise, Haddock with Creamy Yogurt, 108–109
Meal plans
    about, 16, 19
    for families, 28–31
    quick and easy, 20–23
    for weight loss, 24–27
Meatballs
    Lentil "Meat"balls with Basil and Parmesan, 70–71
    Spaghetti and Vegetarian "Meat"balls, 92–93
    Turkey, Apple, and Cranberry Meatballs, 142–143

Meatloaf
    Barbecue-Glazed Meatloaf, 162–163
    Veggie Meatloaf, 86–87
Meats, 10–11. *See also specific*
Mirepoix, 5-Ingredient, 199
Mushrooms
    Beef and Mushroom Burgers, 164–165
    5-Ingredient Mirepoix, 199
    One-Pot Pasta with Ground Turkey
        and Mushroom Sauce, 139

N

Noodles. *See* Pasta and noodles
Nut-free
    Apple Flapjacks, 48
    Avocado-Dill Dressing, 196
    Avocado-Dill Poached Salmon, 114–115
    Baked Salmon with Creamy Cilantro Dressing, 112
    Barbecue-Glazed Meatloaf, 162–163
    Barbecue Pork Chops, 152–153
    Barbecue Turkey Bowls, 146–147
    Beef and Broccoli Stir-Fry, 166–167
    Beef and Mushroom Burgers, 164–165
    Black Bean Fiesta Bowls, 80
    Blueberry-Peach Smoothie, 44
    Butternut Squash and Tomato Soup, 52
    Carrot-Ginger Soup, 55
    Carrot, Mango, and Citrus Smoothie, 45
    Chicken, Lettuce, and Tomato Sandwiches
        with Creamy Cilantro Dressing, 65
    Chicken Parmesan, 136–137
    Chickpea, Kale, and Sweet Potato Bowls, 78
    Chickpea, Lentil, and Avocado Sandwiches, 63
    Chocolate-Avocado Pudding, 178
    Cinnamon Oat and Pear Smoothie, 46
    Cinnamon Toast Oatmeal, 35
    Coconut-Mango Green Smoothie, 47
    Cream of Asparagus Soup, 56
    Creamy Cilantro Dressing, 194
    Crispy Chickpeas, 201
    Cucumber, Tomato, and Basil Salad, 60
    Curried Cauliflower Soup, 54
    Curried Lentil Stew, 83
    Date-Sweetened Barbecue Sauce, 191
    Date-Sweetened Teriyaki Sauce, 190
    Dijon Roasted Chicken with Grits, 132–133
    DIY Taco Seasoning, 198

Nut-free *(continued)*
    Fiesta Chicken Macro Bowls, 124–125
    5-Ingredient Mirepoix, 199
    Foil-Wrapped Tuscan Haddock, 107
    Ginger Pickled Radish, 200
    Green-Powered Smoothie, 42
    Grilled Rosemary Flank Steak with
        Seasoned Farro, 170–171
    Haddock with Creamy Yogurt Mayonnaise, 108–109
    Herbed Chicken with Couscous
        and Spinach, 122–123
    Honey-Glazed Carrots, 204
    Honey-Glazed Pork Chops, 150–151
    Hummus Tabbouleh Wraps, 64
    Italian Wedding Soup, 144–145
    Kale Crisps, 202
    Lemon-Basil Vinaigrette, 192
    Lemon-Blueberry Parfaits, 176
    Lemon-Caper Aïoli, 197
    Lemon-Ricotta Cupcakes, 184
    Lemony Lentil Soup, 53
    Lentil "Meat"balls with Basil and Parmesan, 70–71
    Lightened Beef Stroganoff, 172–173
    Maple-Tahini Brownies, 185
    Mediterranean Bowls, 79
    Mexican-Inspired Tilapia with Bell
        Peppers and Kale, 106
    One-Pot Chicken with Penne and
        Tomatoes, 138
    One-Pot Pasta with Ground Turkey
        and Mushroom Sauce, 139
    One-Pot Taco Shrimp, 99
    Panko-Crusted Chicken with Dipping
        Sauce Trio, 128–129
    Pan-Seared Pork Chops with Kale,
        Corn, and Bell Pepper, 154–155
    Pan-Seared Tilapia over Lemon-
        Parmesan Pasta, 104–105
    Pear, Spinach, and Ricotta Omelet, 38–39
    Peppered Beef Macro Bowls, 168
    Pineapple Chicken, 126–127
    Roasted Veggie Mac-n-Cheese Au Gratin, 90–91
    Sautéed Eggplant with Peppers and Onions, 75
    Seared Fish Tacos with Mango-Lime
        Salsa, 102–103
    Sesame Salmon Protein Bowls, 116–117
    Shrimp and Arugula Salad, 98

    Shrimp and Grits over Collard Greens, 100–101
    Simple Baked Chicken with Potato and
        Green Bean Salad, 130–131
    Smooth Zucchini Soup, 66
    Spaghetti and Vegetarian "Meat"balls, 92–93
    Strawberry-Basil Smoothie, 41
    Stuffed Bell Peppers, 160–161
    Stuffed Eggplant with Savory Vegan Cream, 76–77
    Sweet Potato Medallions, 203
    Tabbouleh Salad with Farro, 58
    Tahini Roasted Salmon with Warm
        Kale Salad, 110–111
    Tamale-Style Grits and Eggs, 37
    Teriyaki Black Bean Burgers, 72–73
    Teriyaki Chicken with Kale Salad and
        Sweet Potato Medallions, 134–135
    Teriyaki Salmon Bowls, 113
    Teriyaki Veggie Stir-Fry, 74
    Tuna Toasts with Lemon-Caper Aïoli, 96
    Turkey Burgers with Creamy
        Cilantro Dressing, 140–141
    Turmeric-Tahini Dressing, 195
    Vegetarian Shepherd's Pie, 88–89
    Veggie Burger Parmesan, 84–85
    Veggie Meatloaf, 86–87
Nuts, 13
    Apple and Walnut Salad over Greens, 62
    Banana-Nut Overnight Oats, 36
    Cashew Chicken, 121
    Coconut-Almond Macaroons, 182–183
    Honey-Almond Energy Bites, 180

Oats
    Banana-Nut Overnight Oats, 36
    Cinnamon Oat and Pear Smoothie, 46
    Cinnamon Toast Oatmeal, 35
    Maple-Date Granola, 40
    Maple-Sesame Oat Cake with
        Blueberry Topping, 186–187
One pot/pan
    Avocado-Dill Dressing, 196
    Baked Salmon with Creamy Cilantro Dressing, 112
    Carrot, Mango, and Citrus Smoothie, 45
    Chicken, Lettuce, and Tomato Sandwiches
        with Creamy Cilantro Dressing, 65
    Chickpea, Kale, and Sweet Potato Bowls, 78

Chocolate-Avocado Pudding, 178
Cinnamon Oat and Pear Smoothie, 46
Creamy Cilantro Dressing, 194
Date-Sweetened Barbecue Sauce, 191
Date-Sweetened Teriyaki Sauce, 190
DIY Taco Seasoning, 198
Ginger Pickled Radish, 200
Green-Powered Smoothie, 42
Honey-Glazed Carrots, 204
Hummus Tabbouleh Wraps, 64
Lemon-Basil Vinaigrette, 192
Lemon-Caper Aïoli, 197
Mediterranean Bowls, 79
One-Pot Chicken with Penne and Tomatoes, 138
One-Pot Pasta with Ground Turkey
    and Mushroom Sauce, 139
Pan-Seared Pork Chops with Kale,
    Corn, and Bell Pepper, 154–155
Peppered Beef Macro Bowls, 168
Pineapple Pork with Roasted Vegetables, 158–159
Sesame Avocado Salad, 57
Sesame Chicken Chopped Salad, 120
Sesame Dressing, 193
Sesame Mandarin and Edamame Salad, 59
Tamale-Style Grits and Eggs, 37
Teriyaki Pork Stir-Fry, 157
Teriyaki Veggie Stir-Fry, 74
Turmeric-Tahini Dressing, 195
Onions
    5-Ingredient Mirepoix, 199
    Sautéed Eggplant with Peppers and Onions, 75
Oranges
    Carrot, Mango, and Citrus Smoothie, 45
    Sesame Mandarin and Edamame Salad, 59

Panko-Crusted Chicken with Dipping
    Sauce Trio, 128–129
Parmesan cheese
    Chicken Parmesan, 136–137
    Lentil "Meat"balls with Basil and
        Parmesan, 70–71
    Pan-Seared Tilapia over Lemon-
        Parmesan Pasta, 104–105
    Veggie Burger Parmesan, 84–85
Pasta and noodles
    Ginger-Soy Noodle Bowls, 82

Lightened Beef Stroganoff, 172–173
One-Pot Chicken with Penne and Tomatoes, 138
One-Pot Pasta with Ground Turkey
    and Mushroom Sauce, 139
Pan-Seared Tilapia over Lemon-
    Parmesan Pasta, 104–105
Roasted Veggie Mac-n-Cheese Au
    Gratin, 90–91
Spaghetti and Vegetarian "Meat"balls, 92–93
Peach Smoothie, Blueberry-, 46
Peanut Butter and Chocolate Chip Cookies, 181
Pears
    Cinnamon Oat and Pear Smoothie, 46
    Pear, Spinach, and Ricotta Omelet, 38–39
Peppered Beef Macro Bowls, 168
Pickled Radish, Ginger, 200
Pineapple
    Pineapple Chicken, 126–127
    Pineapple Pork with Roasted
        Vegetables, 158–159
Pork
    Barbecue Pork Chops, 152–153
    Honey-Glazed Pork Chops, 150–151
    Pan-Seared Pork Chops with Kale,
        Corn, and Bell Pepper, 154–155
    Pineapple Pork with Roasted
        Vegetables, 158–159
    Spicy Chili Pork Bowls, 156
    Teriyaki Pork Stir-Fry, 157
Portion sizing, 3
Potato and Green Bean Salad, Simple
    Baked Chicken with, 130–131
Processed foods, 2, 11, 12–13
Proteins, 8–9
Pudding, Chocolate-Avocado, 178

Quinoa Harvest Bowls, 81

R

Radish, Ginger Pickled, 200
Recipes, about, 15–17
Ricotta cheese
    Lemon-Ricotta Cupcakes, 184
    Pear, Spinach, and Ricotta Omelet, 38–39
Rosemary Flank Steak with Seasoned
    Farro, Grilled, 170–171

S

Salads
 Apple and Walnut Salad over Greens, 62
 Cucumber, Tomato, and Basil Salad, 60
 Sesame Avocado Salad, 57
 Sesame Avocado Salad with Tuna, 97
 Sesame Chicken Chopped Salad, 120
 Sesame Mandarin and Edamame Salad, 59
 Shrimp and Arugula Salad, 98
 Simple Baked Chicken with Potato and
  Green Bean Salad, 130–131
 Steak Salad with Sesame Dressing, 169
 Strawberry-Spinach Salad with
  Lemon-Basil Vinaigrette, 61
 Tabbouleh Salad with Farro, 58
 Tahini Roasted Salmon with Warm
  Kale Salad, 110–111
 Teriyaki Chicken with Kale Salad and
  Sweet Potato Medallions, 134–135
Salmon
 Avocado-Dill Poached Salmon, 114–115
 Baked Salmon with Creamy Cilantro Dressing, 112
 Sesame Salmon Protein Bowls, 116–117
 Tahini Roasted Salmon with Warm
  Kale Salad, 110–111
 Teriyaki Salmon Bowls, 113
Salsa, Seared Fish Tacos with Mango-Lime, 102–103
Sandwiches and wraps
 Blueberry-Basil Avocado Toasts, 34
 Chicken, Lettuce, and Tomato Sandwiches
  with Creamy Cilantro Dressing, 65
 Chickpea, Lentil, and Avocado Sandwiches, 63
 Hummus Tabbouleh Wraps, 64
 Tuna Toasts with Lemon-Caper Aïoli, 96
Sauces
 Date-Sweetened Barbecue Sauce, 191
 Date-Sweetened Teriyaki Sauce, 190
Seasoning, DIY Taco, 198
Seeds, 13
Seltzer water, 12
Sesame. *See also* Tahini
 Maple-Sesame Oat Cake with
  Blueberry Topping, 186–187
 Sesame Avocado Salad, 57
 Sesame Avocado Salad with Tuna, 97
 Sesame Chicken Chopped Salad, 120

 Sesame Dressing, 193
 Sesame Mandarin and Edamame Salad, 59
 Sesame Salmon Protein Bowls, 116–117
 Steak Salad with Sesame Dressing, 169
Shepherd's Pie, Vegetarian, 88–89
Shrimp
 One-Pot Taco Shrimp, 99
 Shrimp and Arugula Salad, 98
 Shrimp and Grits over Collard Greens, 100–101
Sleep, 5
Smoothies, 13
 Blueberry-Peach Smoothie, 44
 Carrot, Mango, and Citrus Smoothie, 45
 Cinnamon Oat and Pear Smoothie, 46
 Coconut-Mango Green Smoothie, 47
 Green-Powered Smoothie, 42
 Mango Cream Smoothie, 43
 Strawberry-Basil Smoothie, 41
Sodas, 12
Sodium, 11
Soups and stews
 Butternut Squash and Tomato Soup, 52
 Carrot-Ginger Soup, 55
 Cream of Asparagus Soup, 56
 Curried Cauliflower Soup, 54
 Curried Lentil Stew, 83
 Italian Wedding Soup, 144–145
 Lemony Lentil Soup, 53
 Smooth Zucchini Soup, 66
Spaghetti and Vegetarian "Meat"balls, 92–93
Spinach
 Herbed Chicken with Couscous
  and Spinach, 122–123
 Pear, Spinach, and Ricotta
  Omelet, 38–39
 Strawberry-Spinach Salad with
  Lemon-Basil Vinaigrette, 61
Steak Salad with Sesame Dressing, 169
Stir-fries
 Beef and Broccoli Stir-Fry, 166–167
 Teriyaki Pork Stir-Fry, 157
 Teriyaki Veggie Stir-Fry, 74
Strawberries
 Strawberries and Cream, 179
 Strawberry-Basil Smoothie, 41
 Strawberry-Spinach Salad with
  Lemon-Basil Vinaigrette, 61

Stress management, 5
Sugars, 10
Sweeteners, 10
Sweet potatoes
    Chickpea, Kale, and Sweet Potato
        Bowls, 78
    Sweet Potato Medallions, 203
    Teriyaki Chicken with Kale Salad and
        Sweet Potato Medallions, 134–135

T

Tabbouleh Salad with Farro, 58
Taco Seasoning, DIY, 198
Tacos with Mango-Lime Salsa,
    Seared Fish, 102–103
Tahini
    Maple-Sesame Oat Cake with
        Blueberry Topping, 186–187
    Maple-Tahini Brownies, 185
    Tahini Roasted Salmon with Warm
        Kale Salad, 110–111
    Turmeric-Tahini Dressing, 195
Tamale-Style Grits and Eggs, 37
Teriyaki
    Date-Sweetened Teriyaki Sauce, 190
    Teriyaki Black Bean Burgers, 72–73
    Teriyaki Chicken with Kale Salad and
        Sweet Potato Medallions, 134–135
    Teriyaki Pork Stir-Fry, 157
    Teriyaki Salmon Bowls, 113
    Teriyaki Veggie Stir-Fry, 74
30-minute meals
    Apple and Walnut Salad over Greens, 62
    Apple Flapjacks, 48
    Avocado-Dill Poached Salmon, 114–115
    Baked Salmon with Creamy Cilantro Dressing, 112
    Barbecue Pork Chops, 152–153
    Barbecue Turkey Bowls, 146–147
    Beef and Broccoli Stir-Fry, 166–167
    Black Bean Fiesta Bowls, 80
    Blueberry-Basil Avocado Toasts, 34
    Carrot, Mango, and Citrus Smoothie, 45
    Cashew Chicken, 121
    Chicken, Lettuce, and Tomato Sandwiches
        with Creamy Cilantro Dressing, 65
    Chicken Parmesan, 136–137
    Chickpea, Kale, and Sweet Potato Bowls, 78

Chickpea, Lentil, and Avocado Sandwiches, 63
Chocolate-Avocado Pudding, 178
Cinnamon Oat and Pear Smoothie, 46
Cinnamon Toast Oatmeal, 35
Coconut-Almond Macaroons, 182–183
Coconut-Mango Green Smoothie, 47
Cream of Asparagus Soup, 56
Dijon Roasted Chicken with Grits, 132–133
Fiesta Chicken Macro Bowls, 124–125
Foil-Wrapped Tuscan Haddock, 107
Ginger-Soy Noodle Bowls, 82
Green-Powered Smoothie, 42
Haddock with Creamy Yogurt Mayonnaise, 108–109
Herbed Chicken with Couscous
    and Spinach, 122–123
Honey-Glazed Pork Chops, 150–151
Hummus Tabbouleh Wraps, 64
Lemon-Ricotta Cupcakes, 184
Lightened Beef Stroganoff, 172–173
Mediterranean Bowls, 79
Mexican-Inspired Tilapia with Bell
    Peppers and Kale, 106
One-Pot Chicken with Penne and Tomatoes, 138
One-Pot Pasta with Ground Turkey
    and Mushroom Sauce, 139
Panko-Crusted Chicken with Dipping
    Sauce Trio, 128–129
Pan-Seared Pork Chops with Kale,
    Corn, and Bell Pepper, 154–155
Pan-Seared Tilapia over Lemon-
    Parmesan Pasta, 104–105
Peanut Butter and Chocolate Chip Cookies, 181
Pear, Spinach, and Ricotta Omelet, 38–39
Pineapple Pork with Roasted
    Vegetables, 158–159
Seared Fish Tacos with Mango-Lime Salsa, 102–103
Sesame Avocado Salad, 57
Sesame Avocado Salad with Tuna, 97
Sesame Chicken Chopped Salad, 120
Sesame Mandarin and Edamame Salad, 59
Sesame Salmon Protein Bowls, 116–117
Shrimp and Arugula Salad, 98
Spicy Chili Pork Bowls, 156
Steak Salad with Sesame Dressing, 169
Strawberry-Spinach Salad with
    Lemon-Basil Vinaigrette, 61
Stuffed Bell Peppers, 160–161

30-minute meals *(continued)*
    Tahini Roasted Salmon with Warm
        Kale Salad, 110–111
    Tamale-Style Grits and Eggs, 37
    Teriyaki Pork Stir-Fry, 157
    Teriyaki Salmon Bowls, 113
    Teriyaki Veggie Stir-Fry, 74
    Tuna Toasts with Lemon-Caper Aïoli, 96
    Turkey, Apple, and Cranberry Meatballs, 142–143
    Turkey Burgers with Creamy
        Cilantro Dressing, 140–141
Tilapia
    Mexican-Inspired Tilapia with Bell
        Peppers and Kale, 106
    Pan-Seared Tilapia over Lemon-
        Parmesan Pasta, 104–105
    Seared Fish Tacos with Mango-Lime Salsa, 102–103
Tomatoes
    Butternut Squash and Tomato Soup, 52
    Chicken, Lettuce, and Tomato Sandwiches
        with Creamy Cilantro Dressing, 65
    Cucumber, Tomato, and Basil Salad, 60
    One-Pot Chicken with Penne and Tomatoes, 138
Tools and equipment, 14–15
Tuna
    Sesame Avocado Salad with Tuna, 97
    Tuna Toasts with Lemon-Caper Aïoli, 96
Turkey, 11
    Barbecue Turkey Bowls, 146–147
    Italian Wedding Soup, 144–145
    One-Pot Pasta with Ground Turkey
        and Mushroom Sauce, 139
    Turkey, Apple, and Cranberry Meatballs, 142–143
    Turkey Burgers with Creamy
        Cilantro Dressing, 140–141
Turmeric-Tahini Dressing, 195

V

Vegan
    Avocado-Dill Dressing, 196
    Banana-Nut Overnight Oats, 36
    Blueberry-Basil Avocado Toasts, 34
    Blueberry-Peach Smoothie, 44
    Carrot, Mango, and Citrus Smoothie, 45
    Chickpea, Kale, and Sweet Potato Bowls, 78
    Chocolate-Avocado Pudding, 178
    Cinnamon Oat and Pear Smoothie, 46

Coconut-Mango Green Smoothie, 47
Crispy Chickpeas, 201
Cucumber, Tomato, and Basil Salad, 60
Curried Cauliflower Soup, 54
Curried Lentil Stew, 83
Date-Sweetened Teriyaki Sauce, 190
DIY Taco Seasoning, 198
5-Ingredient Mirepoix, 199
Ginger Pickled Radish, 200
Green-Powered Smoothie, 42
Hummus Tabbouleh Wraps, 64
Kale Crisps, 202
Lemon-Basil Vinaigrette, 192
Lemony Lentil Soup, 53
Mango Cream Smoothie, 43
Maple-Date Granola, 40
Sautéed Eggplant with Peppers and Onions, 75
Sesame Mandarin and Edamame Salad, 59
Strawberries and Cream, 179
Strawberry-Basil Smoothie, 41
Strawberry-Spinach Salad with
    Lemon-Basil Vinaigrette, 61
Stuffed Eggplant with Savory Vegan Cream, 76–77
Sweet Potato Medallions, 203
Tabbouleh Salad with Farro, 58
Teriyaki Veggie Stir-Fry, 74
Turmeric-Tahini Dressing, 195
Vegetables, 10. *See also specific*
    Pineapple Pork with Roasted Vegetables, 158–159
    Roasted Veggie Mac-n-Cheese Au Gratin, 90–91
    Teriyaki Veggie Stir-Fry, 74
    Veggie Burger Parmesan, 84–85
    Veggie Meatloaf, 86–87
Vegetarian. *See also* Vegan
    Apple and Walnut Salad over Greens, 62
    Apple Flapjacks, 48
    Black Bean Fiesta Bowls, 80
    Carrot-Ginger Soup, 55
    Cheesecake Parfaits, 177
    Chickpea, Lentil, and Avocado Sandwiches, 63
    Cinnamon Toast Oatmeal, 35
    Coconut-Almond Macaroons, 182–183
    Cream of Asparagus Soup, 56
    Creamy Cilantro Dressing, 194
    Date-Sweetened Barbecue Sauce, 191
    Ginger-Soy Noodle Bowls, 82
    Honey-Almond Energy Bites, 180

Honey-Glazed Carrots, 204
Lemon-Blueberry Parfaits, 176
Lemon-Caper Aïoli, 197
Lemon-Ricotta Cupcakes, 184
Lentil "Meat"balls with Basil and Parmesan, 70–71
Maple-Sesame Oat Cake with
    Blueberry Topping, 186–187
Maple-Tahini Brownies, 185
Mediterranean Bowls, 79
Peanut Butter and Chocolate Chip Cookies, 181
Pear, Spinach, and Ricotta Omelet, 38–39
Quinoa Harvest Bowls, 81
Roasted Veggie Mac-n-Cheese Au Gratin, 90–91
Sesame Avocado Salad, 57
Sesame Dressing, 193
Spaghetti and Vegetarian "Meat"balls, 92–93
Tamale-Style Grits and Eggs, 37
Teriyaki Black Bean Burgers, 72–73
Vegetarian Shepherd's Pie, 88–89

Veggie Burger Parmesan, 84–85
Veggie Meatloaf, 86–87

Walnut Salad over Greens, Apple and, 64
Weight loss, 7
Whole foods, 2
Whole grains, 10. *See also specific*
Wraps. *See* Sandwiches and wraps

Yogurt, 12
    Cheesecake Parfaits, 177
    Haddock with Creamy Yogurt Mayonnaise, 108–109
    Lemon-Blueberry Parfaits, 176

Zucchini Soup, Smooth, 52–53

ACKNOWLEDGMENTS

I'd like to thank Briana Millar for her culinary inspiration. Her intuitive cooking skills and joy for cooking have motivated me to make my dishes well crafted and flavorful. I'm lucky to have my personal test-tasters—my husband, JP, and daughters, Ailish and Julia—who have lent their taste buds to this project. A shout-out to my mom, Carol, and sisters, Rhonda and Tova, for supporting my endeavors in cooking and writing. Lastly, I'm grateful for my editor, Reina Glenn, for guiding me to do my best work.

ABOUT THE AUTHOR

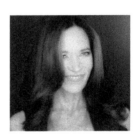 **Lauren O'Connor** is a registered dietitian, yoga instructor, and three-time cookbook author. She offers nutritional counseling and consulting services for individuals and companies nationwide. A member of the Academy of Nutrition and Dietetics (AND) and Food & Culinary Professionals (FCP), she received her master's degree in nutritional sciences from California State University, Los Angeles. As a recipe developer, writer, and credentialed health advocate, she has contributed to national print, radio, and television media.

O'Connor promotes whole-food choices in her plant-based nutritional guidelines, tailoring plans and recipes to best suit her clients' needs. With a specialty in gastroesophageal reflux disease (GERD) management, she promotes dietary and lifestyle practices to improve health outcomes for those with acid-reflux concerns.

CPSIA information can be obtained
at www.ICGtesting.com
Printed in the USA
JSHW020752130621
15830JS00001B/1

9 781648 766244